MW01196791

The *Physician's Guide to Holistic Migraine Relief* series presents...

KETO FOR MIGRAINE

Keys to the Ketogenic Diet for Migraine Sufferers

JOSH TURKNETT, M.D.

A *Healthy Brain Solutions* Publication

Publisher's Note

Library of Congress Cataloging-in-Publication Data on file

To all of my fellow migraine sufferers who have entrusted me with their care and have taught me far more than any textbook ever could.

This book, and the lives it will touch, could not have been possible without you.

CONTENTS

GETTING READY

To help you get the most out of this book, and to further increase your odds of success, my wife Jenny (the mastermind behind all of our recipes) and I have created a **Supplemental Guide to Keto for Migraine**. And it's entirely free to you with your purchase of this book.

I strongly recommend you grab a copy of it, and would recommend doing so now. All you need to do is go to ketoformigraine.com/guide, enter your email, and it shall be delivered to you immediately.

The **Supplemental Guide to Keto for Migraine includes:**

- 30 Keto for Migraine plan recipes

- A one-month meal plan for getting started

- Information and links to all of our favorite keto-related tools and products discussed in the book.

- Our popular "11 Drug Free Strategies For Ending A Migraine"

WELCOME, & THANK YOU

Dear Reader,

All around the world, people are doing what they once thought impossible. What they'd been *told* was impossible.

They're ending their battle with migraines, known around here as "The Beast."

They are leaving their homes no longer checking to be sure they have their migraine medications.

Pill bottles that used to not even last them a month are gathering dust in the medicine cabinet, with expiration dates long past.

Their pharmacists, alarmed by their absence, are filing missing persons reports.

All of this is happening to more and more longtime migraine sufferers each and every day, as word of their success spreads.

How are they doing this?

By ditching the old approach to treating migraine headaches. The old approach that treats migraines as a fate we must accept because of some unlucky bits of DNA. The one in which our only viable options are a handful of drugs.

The one where all we're given is a squirt gun, while The Beast has a nuclear missile.

Worse yet, by ignoring root causes and disrupting health, it's an approach that makes our migraines *worse* over time.

They are achieving the "impossible" by abandoning that old and ineffective approach and replacing it with a new and vastly improved one. One that doesn't involve pills.

They are throwing out the naive and outdated idea that we can outsmart our bodies with a single magic pill. In its place, they are adopting an approach that taps into the body's infinite wisdom to solve its own problems. One that recognizes that the body is an interconnected system. One that works with our body, not against it.

One that recognizes that our genes are neither our fate nor the primary driver of health.

How has this movement grown? Through people just like you putting this holistic approach into action, providing living proof to others what's possible when you do.

For a long time, it seemed like we were stuck, and that we'd be stuck forever. For a long time, I had nothing to offer my migraine patients, and it seemed I never would. As a physician committed to relieving suffering and as a migraine sufferer myself, this was a demoralizing situation.

Now, nothing could be further from the truth.

Yet, there are far too many people still suffering. But each day more and more people are reached, thanks to folks just like you. People taking action, and achieving results that speak for themselves.

And it hasn't come from people preaching from on high, and it hasn't come from the "experts." Instead, it has come from those leading by quiet example. With results like these, there's no need to shout.

This is why I know this movement will only continue. That even though so many lives have already been impacted, this is only the beginning.

I'm so excited you're here. And I'm so excited for you, because I know what lies in store.

So let's do this.

Let's go Slay the Beast!

Dr. T

p.s. - To get a glimpse of what's in store, and to get a jolt of inspiration, check out our success story interviews at ketoformigraine.com/stories.

p.p.s - A chapter by chapter list of references for this book, including links to the primary sources, can be found at ketoformigraine.com/references.

WHO AM I?

If you're like me, you might make your way through an entire book without even knowing the name of the author. Much less his or her reasons for writing the book. Those pieces of information aren't essential for your reading experience.

In the case of this book, however, I think knowing my background and reasons for writing this book *are* useful information and will enhance your experience in reading this book.

So allow me to briefly share the story of how I got here, writing these words that you're now reading.

If you'd told me ten years ago that I'd be writing books about migraines, and be regarded as a leading expert on diet and lifestyle strategies for ending them, I wouldn't have believed you.

Yes, I've personally suffered from migraines for my whole life. Yes, I'm a neurologist and migraine expert. From that standpoint, my writing books for migraine sufferers doesn't seem far fetched.

But ten years ago, I didn't think there was much to say on the subject. I knew all there was to know about migraines and how to treat them. That was my area of professional expertise, after all.

My patients received the best care that modern medicine had to offer, as did I. **We all wanted something much better, but it seemed a long way off.** Progress in the world of migraine treatments, like so many areas of medicine, was agonizingly slow.

Actually, to many of us, myself included, it felt like things were going *backward*. It seemed like, if anything, what we were doing was making matters worse.

And then I inadvertently stumbled upon a way out — a path to migraine freedom previously unbeknownst to me or my colleagues.

So there I was, possessed of this knowledge that I knew could transform the lives of migraineurs everywhere. Knowledge that few others possessed. Clearly I had no choice but to share what I'd learned. Not if I wanted to sleep at night with a clear conscience, at least.

Since that first book came out, the impact has been beyond my wildest dreams. Our migraine community now spans over 30 countries.

And every day, we receive new stories from all over the world of people ending their migraine battles after years of struggle. After years of trying every single thing out there. Experiencing this after having already resigned themselves to the idea that such a thing wasn't possible. After accepting that chronic migraines were their fate.

In that time, we've learned so much. **That includes the lessons learned in helping thousands of migraineurs implement a ketogenic diet.**

As you'll learn in this book, keto can be an extraordinarily powerful weapon for the migraineur - when it's used wisely. Not all keto roads lead where the migraineur wants to go.

I've learned the common mistakes. I've made those mistakes myself.

I've learned how keto can make migraineurs' lives better. And how it can make them worse.

So, here I find myself, nearly a decade later, in a very similar situation, with a story about the ketogenic diet for migraine that really only I can tell. Because this is such new terrain, I imagine I've worked with more people implementing keto for migraine than anyone else on the planet, which means that I also now possess a large body of hard-won practical knowledge.

Knowledge that I know can spell the difference between disappointment at yet another failed migraine treatment or a life transformed beyond anything you could've possibly imagined.

That's too important not to share.

ABOUT THE PHYSICIANS GUIDE TO HOLISTIC MIGRAINE RELIEF SERIES (OR WHAT DOES HOLISTIC REALLY MEAN?)

"The art of medicine consists of amusing the patient while nature takes care of the disease."

- Voltaire

"The human body is the most extraordinary self righting machine".

- Dr. Joel Fleischman

✱ ✱ ✱

What does the word "holistic" mean, exactly?

It's a word that gets thrown around a lot in the realm of health. But its meaning is often a little fuzzy, and the way it's used not always consistent. Since this book is part of the *Physicians Guide To Holistic Migraine Relief* series, it's probably a good idea we sorted that out!

Sometimes "holistic" is used to describe a "natural" approach to health, which itself can mean all manner of things.

Sometimes it's used to describe an approach that's more humane, that treats people like complete human beings with hopes, dreams, fears, and desires, rather than as objects with specific problems to be fixed. Something more than "the chronic migraine in exam room 3."

Sometimes it's used to indicate a wide-reaching, multi-disciplinary approach to health.

These are all right in their own way, but it goes deeper than that.

As I said, this book is part of the *Physicians Guide To Holistic Migraine Relief* series. I'm an M.D., and very few of my colleagues would use the word "holistic" to describe the kind of medicine they practice.

Over the years, western medicine has become increasingly specialized. Specialists don't concern themselves with the big picture, just a tiny slice of it. The rest of the picture is irrelevant to our purposes.

Our collective project in biology and medicine over the past half-century or so has been to *reduce* the workings of the body to its constituent elements (organs, then cells, then molecules, then DNA, and so on). We thought that doing so would unlock the secrets of health and disease. This process of studying a phenomenon by breaking it down into its smaller components is known as "reductionism."

The problem, however, is that you can't understand the workings of the body and brain by studying its pieces in isolation.

Everything is connected.

Breaking things into parts can help keep stuff organized, especially in a system as complex as the human body, but that compartmentalization doesn't reflect how things actually work.

Like the parable of the blind man and the elephant, when you focus your attention on only a small slice of the picture, you fail to recognize what it is you're seeing.

It's crucial, then, for you to understand what "holistic" means. In almost every way, it's the polar opposite of the standard reductionist approach of western medicine. That includes the standard approach to migraines that you're probably familiar with, and which likely informs your own thinking on the subject.

But, truly understanding what a holistic approach is, and all that it entails, is critical to your success. So let's define it clearly.

In a reductionist approach to health, we're looking for a *single cause* for our problem (a "smoking gun")

In a holistic approach to health, we recognize there are many causes and factors since nothing in the body works in isolation.

In a reductionist approach to health, we try to find the solution to our problems (" we know best").

In a holistic approach to health, we try to provide the body what it needs to solve its problems ("the body knows best").

In a reductionist approach to health, our primary treatments are pharmaceuticals, which *disrupt* what the body is trying to do (because we believe doing so will move things in a better direction).

In a holistic approach to health, we look for ways to *activate, support, and amplify* our body's ability to heal itself and thrive.

In a reductionist approach to health, we view health and disease as binary, either/or, states (i.e., you're either healthy or you're sick).

In a holistic approach to health, we recognize that health and disease is a continuum.

In a reductionist approach to health, we believe we can find the one thing that will fix what ails us.

In a holistic approach to health, we recognize that there are no silver bullets. We achieve better health and relief from health problems through the synergistic combination of all of our health behaviors. It's no one thing that helps us, it's *all the things*.

THE GREAT STAGNATION

Part of why I chose to enter the field of neurology after graduating medical school in 2001 was because, like so many, I believed we were on the cusp of some major breakthroughs in our ability to treat neurological conditions.

Neuroscience was blossoming, fueled by intense interest in the potential of better understanding our brain and new technologies for doing so. The sense of possibility was intoxicating.

In 2000, I asked a prominent Alzheimer's researcher how long he thought it would be until we had a drug that would cure the disease. His response?

10 years.

The reality of what has *actually* happened since then could not be more different. Or disappointing.

It's nearly twenty years later as I'm writing this, and not only is there not a cure for Alzheimer's, **there isn't even a single treatment that's marginally better than what was available in 2000,**

when he made that prediction.

Our failure to find effective medicines isn't just limited to Alzheimer's, unfortunately. In my entire career, we've made no significant breakthroughs in any of the diseases neurologists treat. The last significant one was the release of sumatriptan for migraine in 1991 (and given that it has also fueled an epidemic of rebound headaches, some would argue that it wasn't a breakthrough).

If we remove sumatriptan from the list, we have to go all the way back to the mid 20th Century for the last treatment breakthrough.

For well over a half-century, we've made virtually no progress in the treatment of neurological diseases, nor have we made any significant progress in virtually every chronic disease of our times. No progress since the time before cell phones. Before the internet. Before personal computers. Before MRIs. Before CT scans.

I became increasingly unsettled by this fact during the course of my own career. What on earth was going on here?

How could it be that in spite of the incredible technological progress in other areas of human life, in spite of the billions upon billions of dollars spent researching new treatments, and in spite of incredible progress in our understanding of human biology, we had nothing to show for it?

How could it be that in spite of all of that, I had no new options I could offer my patients? Why were most of the treatments my colleagues and I still using nearly centuries old?

Patients came to me, expecting I could alleviate their suffering. Given what they'd heard from the media, they thought that modern medicine was like their smartphones, with new and improved treatments coming fast and furious.

Not only did I not have the tools I needed to fulfill my mission to relieve suffering, in many cases, the ones I did have just made matters worse.

I now wholeheartedly believe that the absence of a holistic perspective is the reason we're in this predicament. Not only does this make sense from a philosophical perspective, but it also makes sense from a practical one as well.

Why? Because by adopting a holistic approach to migraine care, I've been able to help those I work with experience results far surpassing any I ever achieved using the tools of reductionism (listen to any of the success stories at ketoformigraine.com/stories - the results they've achieved are unheard of using the traditional approach to migraine care).

The same can be said of other providers who've achieved similar results using a holistic approach with other notoriously difficult to treat chronic conditions.

For many years, the future seemed bleak. Cold hard reality had dashed our once unbridled enthusiasm. The therapeutic revolution in pharmaceutical treatments had not materialized, nor did it appear it ever would.

Yet, nearly twenty years since that researcher made his failed prediction about a drug cure for Alzheimer's, I am more optimistic than ever.

The solutions to our problems are emerging. They just look different than what we were expecting.

We thought those solutions were going to come in the form of drugs. That was a naive fantasy.

It turns out the solution was under our noses all along. It just requires us to let go of what hasn't worked. And it requires letting go of the attitudes and mindsets that go with the old and broken way.

My hope is that these books will not only lead you to the path of migraine freedom, but to an entirely new and improved way of looking at health, and a future of thriving and well-being you never dared to dream possible.

BE THE BAMBOO

The power of the mind never ceases to amaze me. The idea that the thoughts in our head can influence every single aspect of our health seems implausible.

Even though I've seen the research, and even though I understand the neurobiology that makes this possible, I still find this magical. Though I can appreciate intellectually that it's an illusion, it still doesn't change the fact that it *feels* like my mind exists in another dimension from my body. It *feels* like one shouldn't be able to impact the other.

And yet, if we accept the illusion and fail to appreciate the incredible impact our mind has over our health, then we not only undermine our path to health and wellness, but we fail to take advantage of **our single greatest tool in our quest for a long life well lived.**

Because it is so surprisingly powerful, and because its influence is so often overlooked, I talk about the mind and mindset quite a lot. It's so important in fact that there will be an entire book in the *Physicians Guide To Holistic Migraine Relief* series dedicated to the topic.

Mindset is about the stories we tell ourselves about our lives. The fact that we get to *choose* those stories is one of the greatest gifts of all.

One of my favorite stories is about bamboo. It comes from one of my favorite books, *Chop Wood Carry Water*, which is all about the key mindsets for success. It is perhaps the single best story for understanding what it means to think holistically, and how different that is from the way we've been conditioned to think about health and illness.

THE STORY OF BAMBOO

To grow bamboo, you must first plant the seed. Then, you must water it every day.

Yet, for five years, nothing happens. Correction, for five years, nothing happens *above the surface*. Nothing happens that you can *see* with your own eyes.

Underground, however, much *is* happening. The bamboo is building a dense root structure. And when, after five years it finally emerges from the ground, it shoots up to over ninety feet tall in just six weeks.

In these days of quick fixes, withering attention spans, and instant gratification, most people wouldn't have the patience to grow bamboo. Furthermore, even if they did all the right things to help it grow, they'd be inclined to erroneously conclude, based on the lack of observable results, that their efforts were for naught. That they must've planted a bad seed, or watered it too much or too little.

Not only would they never end up growing any bamboo, **but their ideas about what it takes to grow it would be entirely wrong.**

The reason the story of bamboo is such an instructive metaphor is because I've seen this same exact story time and again working with people to implement a holistic approach to migraine relief. Day by day they apply the various components of the plan, establishing the habits and behaviors that we know are key to success, that strengthen the 3 Pillars of Protection against migraine (if you are unfamiliar with the "3 Pillars," we'll cover those later in this book).

Day by day, they start to feel a little better, but seldom are their results immediate. Depending on where they started from, the initial period can be rocky.

Many times I have to encourage them to focus on the process, and provide reassurance that they're on the right track (in fact, the reason I publish so many success stories is to help people persist in the face of perceived setbacks).

Until one day....BAM! Seemingly overnight, things are much better.

So many people I've worked with can look back and identify this precise moment when everything changed, when they knew that they had turned a corner, and could see their efforts bearing serious fruits.

Like the bamboo growing 90 feet in 6 weeks.

In contrast, let's consider the approach that has predominated in Western medicine for almost a century now:

You have a problem, and you go to the doctor. The doctor makes a diagnosis and gives you a prescription that's intended to fix the problem. **Taking this one thing will make you better.**

That's all well and good if your problem is caused by *one thing*, and if you have a medicine that targets *that one thing*.

Problem is, that's not the case with migraines. Nor is it the case with virtually every other chronic condition we doctors see these days.

Which is precisely why we've failed at treating these conditions. And it's precisely why you're holding this book in your hands, still in search of a *real* solution.

But that kind of silver bullet thinking is so pervasive, it's very easy to lapse into it without realizing it. We donate to fund-raisers to find "a cure." We pour trillions of dollars into research to find a miracle drug. We go to the doctor with the naive expectation of getting that *one* prescription that will fix us.

Because silver bullet thinking surrounds us all the time, it's easy for it to influence our thoughts and behaviors without us realizing it. Yet, it stands in direct contrast to a holistic approach to health. And if it continues to influence your thoughts and behaviors, it will continue to stand in your way of success.

I commonly see people who are implementing a holistic approach with a reductionist, silver bullet, mindset. I'd venture to say it's the norm, in fact.

They try one thing for a little while and see what happens. If it works, they keep doing it. If it doesn't, they discard it and move to the next. It's the right idea but the wrong *execution.*

So what can we learn from the story of bamboo about the keys to success with a holistic approach?

There are 3 key lessons we can learn from the story of bamboo:

1) When you are nurturing and supporting the body, great things will happen beneath the surface, even if you can't see it with your own eyes.

2) It's never any *one thing* that produces the results we seek, but the synergistic combination of many things.

3) The results we seek often appear to occur suddenly. While this may give the impression that our improvement occurred overnight, the reality is that everything we did leading up to that point was ne-

cessary to achieve it.

CHAPTER 1: FINDING YOUR PATH

***WHAT YOU'LL LEARN IN THIS CHAPTER:** The recent explosion in popularity of the ketogenic diet is a mixed blessing for migraineurs, as the most commonly found versions of the ketogenic diet are not tailored to the migraine brain.*

In this chapter, you'll learn how this book will allow you to avoid the common mistakes migraineurs make when "going keto."

Back in February of 2016, I wrote the following in a blog post on The Migraine Miracle website: "I have a prediction. You're going to start hearing a LOT more about ketones and the ketogenic diet in the next decade or two."

I can say that again! While I was right that the ketogenic diet was ultimately going to explode in popularity, I was wrong in my estimate of how long that would take to happen.

As I said, that was February of 2016, about three and a half years ago. As hard as it is to believe now, at the time I wrote it, it was safe to assume that virtually nobody reading that post had ever even heard the word ketogenic diet, ketosis, or "keto." Amazing.

To say a lot has changed since then would be the understatement of the year.

And this wasn't just limited to the general public who was unfamiliar with the ketogenic diet. If I'd brought up the topic of ketosis to one of my physician colleagues, they'd more than likely have mistakenly thought I was talking about ketoacidosis. Then they would've proceeded to respond with misplaced concern about its dangers. Now that whole scenario seems quaint (though doctors, unfortunately, remain mostly ignorant on the subject of keto).

These days, *everyone* is talking about the ketogenic diet. I can barely go a single day without seeing or hearing something about it. At my last visit to the grocery store, there was not one but two different magazine covers in the check out aisle prominently advertising their keto articles inside. Keto sells.

It even has its own language. Eating a ketogenic diet is simply known as "going keto," a convenient shorthand that I'll also use throughout this book. In the three years since I made the aforementioned prediction, we've reached the point where if you haven't heard of keto, you risk being accused of living under a rock.

Now, why was I confident enough to make such a bold prediction back then? How did I know it was only a matter of time before the ketogenic diet exploded in popularity?

Number one, because I knew what it could do. I'd witnessed firsthand the transformative impact of the ketogenic diet. And I'd experienced that transformation myself. Nothing is more convincing than results.

Results speak for themselves.

Furthermore, there was a growing body of research - some of which we'll touch on in this book - showing a range of impressive and wide-ranging health benefits. Benefits the likes of which we physicians have not been able to achieve with pharmaceuticals, the traditional tools of our trade.

I also knew that Fat Phobia, that wretched mental affliction of the 20th Century, was on its last legs. For decades, the general public was wrongly advised (by health authorities, myself included!) to avoid dietary fat, especially the kind found in animal foods. As we'll discuss, that's an idea that can no longer be defended.

And the availability of information made possible by the digital age means that the truth about it can no longer be obscured or hidden.

What's so tragic is that we've known for a long time that a ketogenic diet was a powerful therapeutic weapon. The only reason it's been locked away for so long is because of our misguided and misplaced fear of fat. Now that those fears are evaporating, the floodgates have opened. The flood is now upon us, so it's time to learn how to swim!

SO WHY ANOTHER KETO BOOK?

Perhaps by now you've also heard that the ketogenic diet is helpful for migraines. Perhaps you've heard some of the incredible and inspiring stories I've shared on the Migraine Miracle website and Migraine Miracle Moment podcast. Stories from those who are now headache free after decades of daily migraine, and decades of one failed treatment after another.

But if keto is everywhere now, if you can't escape a trip to the grocery store without having multiple keto-related articles at your disposal, then why this book?

Can't you just grab one of those keto guides in the check out aisle, or sit down with your good friend Dr. Google, type in "keto diet recipes," and get crackin'?

I imagine you know where this is going.

Keto's insanely rapid rise to prominence is a double-edged sword. On the one hand, I'm thrilled at the insane popularity of the ketogenic diet, for several reasons. For one, it means people are starting to wake up to the idea that what we eat is arguably the single most powerful tool we have over our health. That what we eat not only helps to keep us healthy, but that it is **also a powerful therapeutic weapon, vastly superior to to any prescription pharmaceutical**.

Trust me, I know.

It also means that Fat Phobia is finally becoming a thing of the past. As I've already discussed, were it not for the wrongful vilification of fat, especially saturated fat, ketogenic diets would've likely been a commonplace medical therapy for the past century.

But the darker side of that insane popularity is that, for the opportunist looking to make a quick buck, keto is a gold mine. Keto is already big business, with new "keto products" coming out seemingly every day. And commercialization almost always ends up obscuring the truth.

We live in a strange time. On the one hand, we now have access to a ridiculous amount of information. We can carry around virtually the entire store of human knowledge on a device that fits in our pocket. Such is the glory of living in the information age.

It's that very access to accurate information that's curing us of Fat Phobia, which paved the way for keto to spread like wildfire.

Yet, it would be just as accurate to say we're *also* living in the *mis*information age. Never in history have we had to contend with so much misinformation. In the old days, when there were barriers to publishing, you could be reasonably certain that the author and editors of whatever book you read at least attempted to print what was true.

Nowadays, all bets are off. By and large, those truth-preserving safeguards don't exist on the internet.

On the internet, there's no such assurance that what you read is rooted in any scientific evidence whatsoever. You're left to figure that out for yourself. Worse yet, we know there are plenty of folks who make a living off of publishing misinformation on the internet.

Ultimately, people make money on what generates clicks, or what attracts eyeballs, regardless of whether it's accurate. And there's probably no subject where there's more misinformation than on the topic of health.

As I said, I know firsthand what keto can do. I've helped thousands of migraineurs put it to use in the past few years with incredible results, and I want every migraine sufferer to have the chance to experience that. As a neurologist and migraine sufferer, I feel obligated to get good information on keto for my fellow migraineurs out into the world. I know how many still desperately need it.

So first and foremost, I want the keto movement to continue to grow. And I want more lives to be transformed by it. That won't happen if we allow the quick-buck-seeking opportunists to control the keto conversation.

But the other equally if not more important reason for writing this book is that the relationship between keto and migraines is a unique one. One thing I've learned over the past several years working with thousands of migraine sufferers going keto is that all ketogenic diets are not created equal.

This isn't just a general book about keto. Instead, it's a book **written specifically for the migraine sufferer who's decided to**

go keto.

As we'll discuss in this book, there is no single ketogenic diet. While it's true that the body can only make ketones under certain conditions, it's also true that there are an endless number of ways you could eat to make that happen.

The presence of ketones in the brain seems to do great things for a migraineur; however, that's not the only thing changing when you start eating a ketogenic diet. Far from it. And when adopting a ketogenic diet, we must be mindful of all the factors that matter to the migraineur.

Without being mindful of those factors, it's entirely possible to eat a version of the ketogenic diet that makes migraines worse. And getting worse is not an uncommon outcome in those who head to the wild west of the web to plot their keto course.

I've seen this story play out so many times now, with increasing frequency as "keto" continues to grow in popularity. A migraineur hears that keto can be helpful, decides to take the plunge, collecting all manner of keto resources from the internet and beyond. And then he or she is defeated when it doesn't help, or makes their migraines worse.

Meanwhile, in helping thousands of migraineurs implement the ketogenic diet, we've learned a lot about the factors that determine success or failure. So it became increasingly clear that, in light of the burgeoning keto craze, this information needed to get out. **Migraineurs needed their own guide to keto to help them avoid all the common pitfalls, and maximize their chances of success.**

Suffice it to say that there are many things that matter a lot to the migraineur that your average person doing keto (usually to help them lose weight) doesn't need to worry about. The objective isn't merely to stimulate nutritional ketosis but to do so in a way that's a net benefit to our health and our heads.

And I imagine there are two kinds of people who will benefit from what's included in these pages.

The first kind are those of you who are using keto as a beast-slaying weapon. You've been inspired by the incredible results others have had using it, and you'd like to experience that for yourself! So the last thing I want is for you to go down this road, to commit to the effort it takes to go keto, only for it to either have no impact on your migraines or, even worse, make the Beast stronger.

As I said, there are a limitless number of paths to ketosis. If that's why you're here, then I want to help ensure that the path you take enables you to make the most of all of the beast-slaying benefits. And I certainly don't want you heading down any of the roads that lead you straight to the Beast's lair.

We've learned so much about keto and migraines these past few years. Much of what we've learned has come from us making our fair share of mistakes. Mistakes that you now won't be making!

So if you're reading this book because you want to harness the Beast Slaying benefits of a ketogenic diet, then this book is definitely for you.

On the other hand, maybe you're here for additional reasons.

Maybe you've heard others raving about how much better they feel overall since going keto. You've heard them rave about how much more energy they have, or how much more clearly they can think, and you want to know what all the fuss is about.

Or maybe you've been told your blood sugar is trending towards the diabetic range, and you want to reverse that trend, like so many have now done.

Or maybe you want to use it to shed some unwanted body fat (its success as a weight-loss tool is the main reason why keto has become so insanely popular).

Or maybe you have a family history of Alzheimer's or Parkinson's, and have heard about its great promise in both preventing and treating those conditions.

The point is that there are many reasons beyond migraine protection for dipping a toe in keto. Personally, I think that cycling in and out of nutritional ketosis should be considered a foundational part of a healthy lifestyle. It's something that I recommend to friends and family, regardless of whether they have migraines or any other conditions that nutritional ketosis has been shown to help.

The most significant benefits of the ketogenic diet may lie in the chronic diseases it can help us *prevent,* giving us the best chance of a long life well-lived.

But if you suffer from migraines, you surely don't want to go keto if it's going to make your migraines worse. On the contrary, you'd just assume reap all those other benefits and have fewer visits from the Beast while you're at it. Win-win.

If so, this book is for you, too.

SECOND TIMER?

I imagine there are some of you reading this who've done keto before. Maybe you had some success. Maybe not. And maybe in light of that, you're a little bit apprehensive about trying it again, wondering if this time will be any different. I get it.

There are at least a couple of good reasons to give it another go.

First and foremost, as I've already discussed, is the fact that **not all keto is created equal.** Some ways of doing keto can help migraines. Some can hurt.

The way I see most people doing keto these days is not something I'd recommend for migraineurs, given that it's more likely to make them worse than better. And of course, we'll talk more about why that is, and what a migraineur-friendly version of keto looks like.

The second reason is that timing matters. One of the most important lessons I've learned in the past several years is that the road to recovery on the Migraine Miracle plan is a progression. Things we do impact us differently depending on where we are along that progression, a topic we'll also discuss in more depth.

We naturally think of ourselves as the same person from day to day. It seems that way to us.

But the reality is much different. **The reality is we are *literally* always changing**.

You are not the same biological being from one day to the next. You aren't even the same entity from one minute to the next.

Your skin cells last about 20 days on average. The cells that line your small intestine last about three. You are physically rebuilding yourself each and every day. You are switching on and switching off different genes all the time.

With this state of constant change comes great opportunity, as we can profoundly shape these changes by the life we lead. Change is the only constant when it comes to the human body, which explains why something that may have not had much impact today can have a radically different impact tomorrow. That includes the impact of keto.

A REQUEST

"The man who tries methods, ignoring principles, is sure to have trouble."

- Harrington Emerson

I would strongly encourage you to read this book in its entirety. I've purposefully distilled the topic down to the essentials to help ensure that you do so.

Resist the temptation to jump straight to the chapter on how to go keto.

After all, I could've just published a book of keto recipes and called it a day.

Why didn't I? I could give a multitude of reasons, but it ultimately boils down to the fact that I want you to succeed. I want to give you the greatest chance of slaying The Beast once and for all.

And, having worked with thousands of migraineurs over the years, I've come to understand the recipe for success. Just knowing the rules isn't part of that recipe. That recipe includes not only an understanding of what to do, but *why you're doing it.*

Many people come just wanting to know the rules. "Just tell me what to eat," "Just give me a list of foods."

I understand where this comes from. It *seems* like that should be all you'd need.

Yet, every time I begrudgingly complied with that request, I regretted it later. Because those I did this for didn't end up succeeding, as I feared. And the whole point of the work I do in writing this book, and in working with patients, is to give you the best chance of success.

I don't want you just to know the "rules." I want you to understand the reasons behind them. I want you to understand the underlying *principles*. While rules are circumstantial and situational, principles are not.

I can't cover every possible scenario or situation you may encounter. If you only have a set of rules, you'll have no way to decide for yourself how to handle those situations when they arise.

If all you have is a set of specific rules to follow, you are dependent, at the mercy of whoever is writing those rules.

If you understand the fundamental principles, then you are in charge, you are empowered, you have the knowledge you need to be successful no matter what life throws your way.

My work isn't done until I've made myself obsolete.

KEYS FROM CHAPTER 1:

1) The ketogenic diet has recently exploded in popularity, because of the eradication of Fat-Phobia, and because it works incredibly well.

2) The ketogenic diet can do great things for the brain, including the brains of migraine sufferers. Yet, not all ketogenic diets are created equal, so we want to ensure that we adopt a version that helps, not hurts.

3) This book will review all that we've learned over the past several years in helping thousands of migraineurs around the world implement a version that helps.

4) Understanding the principles behind the Keto for Migraine plan, which are described in this book, is essential for your success.

CHAPTER 2: THE TRAGIC TALE OF KETO

WHAT YOU'LL LEARN IN THIS CHAPTER: In this chapter, you'll learn why, despite its tremendous promise in treating neurological conditions, clinicians abandoned the ketogenic diet for nearly a century.

You'll learn what the scientific evidence says about how saturated fat in the diet impacts your heart health, including how to respond to friends, family, and even medical professionals who worry about you eating "too much fat."

In the first large scale study of its kind, researchers placed 50 patients with intractable migraines on a ketogenic diet.

The patients selected for this study were considered to be representative of the worst cases of migraines. They had exhausted every available medical and surgical treatment. They were, in the words of the study's authors, "desperate and willing to attempt any procedure, regardless of the effort involved."

The study was a resounding success.

Migraines resolved entirely in 14 subjects. An additional 29 experienced significant reductions either in the intensity or frequency of their migraines.

Of the eleven who did not improve, only two actually maintained ketosis during the study, and did so for only a short while. In other words, **the best predictor of success was whether or not the subjects stuck to the diet**.

Impressive results, right? Migraines vanishing altogether in almost a third of subjects who were considered the worst of the worst cases. Any drug that could produce those results would make billions.

But there's one big problem with this study.

It was published in 1930.

What happened, you ask? How on earth is it possible that you are only now, nearly a century later, learning about the benefits of a ketogenic diet for migraine.

Great question.

You can blame the "Great Fat Scare" of the 20th Century, and its wretched offspring, Fat Phobia.

In one of the most tragic tales in the history of science, in the mid 20th Century we - by "we" I mean the scientific community and those whom it influenced - made an epic blunder.

The details of that wrong turn and the subsequent fallout have been extensively documented elsewhere, so I'll just paint the big picture.

Around the middle of the 20th Century, a scientist had a hunch that dietary fat was the cause of heart disease, specifically of the artery-clogging plaques that ultimately result in heart attacks, as well as strokes. This hunch was based on some research he'd done feeding rabbits a high-fat diet, along with epidemiological studies on the rates of heart disease in different countries.

Now, there's nothing wrong with this story at this point. Almost everything we now consider established truths in science once started as hunches. But hunches aren't supposed to become accepted truths until lots of experiments have been done to confirm those hunches.

That's because the vast majority of hunches turn out to be wrong. In fact, many would argue that the primary job of science is to disprove hunches. Because if you try *really* hard to disprove your hunches through experiments, and you're unable to do so, then you've increased the odds that your hunch is correct.

The problem with this story about the fat-causes-heart-disease hunch is that that's not what happened. At all.

What happened instead was that, in 1977, the hunch that dietary fat was the cause of cardiovascular disease ended up being written into US dietary guidelines. Guidelines written not by scientists, but lawmakers.

That move allowed a hunch about fat causing heart disease to leapfrog the usual vetting process for hunches. Overnight, the hunch became dogma.

At the time, many in the scientific community were alarmed. They thought that telling millions of people how to eat based on an untested hunch was irresponsible.

This new but unsupported dogma that "fat is bad, sugar is just a harmless empty calorie" story was great for the sugar industry, however. The sugar lobby wielded its considerable financial might and political influence to suppress any evidence suggesting the "fat causes heart disease" hunch was wrong, and to discredit or better yet sink the careers of scientists who dared challenge it.

That effort included secretly paying off some of the most high profile researchers in the field of nutrition at the world's most prestigious academic institutions.

Because animal fat, which is higher in saturated fat, was singled out as the primary fat of concern, cardiologists began advising their patients to use things like soybean, canola, and safflower oil instead of animal fats. Restaurant chains capitalized on this health fad by cooking with these oils. These factory-made fats eventually made their way into virtually every processed food on the grocery shelf.

All of this had an enormous impact on our per capita consumption of soybean oil, which from 1909 to 1999, increased 1000%.

That increase is a cause of great concern to many, myself included. When eaten, these fats are incorporated into the membranes of our cells, taking up permanent residence, and forever altering their structure and function. And there's a good reason to believe that this significant increase in consumption of these oils has played a central role in fueling many of the chronic diseases that are so common today.

Excess fats of this kind, through their impact on specific molecules, promote systemic inflammation. The kind of inflammation that lies at the root of virtually every chronic disease - from Alzheimer's to arthritis.

An Astonishing "Discovery"

To get an idea of just how damaging a mistake this has been, consider the tale of the Minnesota Coronary Experiment (MCE). The MCE was a clinical trial designed to test the hunch that animal fat caused heart disease, and that replacing animal fat with vegetable fat would protect people against it.

A randomized clinical trial (RCT) like this is considered the "gold standard" in medical research. Because RCTs are so challenging to conduct for diet studies, they are rarely done. Most nutrition research instead uses low-quality epidemiological studies - the exact kind of research that the dietary fat-heart disease hunch had been based on. The Minnesota Coronary Experiment offered a chance to finally put that hunch to the test.

The study, which took place from 1968 to 1973 included over 9,000 people over 5 years, and involved 6 mental hospitals and nursing homes (controlled diet studies can only really be conducted in institutionalized populations, which is why they're rarely performed). In the study, the intervention group received a low-fat diet and had their foods cooked in vegetable oil (corn oil in this case).

The control group had their food cooked in mostly animal fat.

What happened?

In those who ate the lower-fat diet with vegetable oil in place of animal fat, cholesterol did go down. The only problem? More of them died. **Those who cut animal fat from their diet were 22% more likely to die** during the study period.

A similar study known as the Sydney Diet Heart Study was performed from 1966 to 1973. Here, the intervention group had their animal fat replaced by safflower oil.

What happened?

The same thing. Eating less animal fat and more vegetable oil lowered the subjects' cholesterol. But, more of those subjects died.

Not only did these studies disprove the hunch that animal fat caused heart disease, and the hunch that high cholesterol causes heart disease, they also showed that using vegetable oil instead of animal fat was dangerous.

Hold on a minute, you say.

If, in 1973, we knew that eating less animal fat and more vegetable oil made you more likely to die, then why on earth did lawmakers publish guidelines in 1977 telling people to do just that?

Because the MCE study wasn't published until 2016 (similarly, the Sydney study wasn't published until 2013)!

For reasons nobody may ever know (though I'll allow you to speculate freely), the data was locked away in a basement for four decades after it was collected. Hard to fathom why that would happen given what a massive and expensive undertaking it had been.

And it's hard to even comprehend or compute the full scope of damage caused by The Great Fat Scare. It led to a dramatic rise in our collective consumption of toxic vegetable and seed oils. It led to an enormous increase in our consumption of sugar, with the emergence of an entire industry dedicated to providing foods low in fat and high in refined carbohydrates, fueling our growing epidemic of diabetes and obesity.

And it led to erroneous beliefs about fat and cholesterol that still linger. To this day, most people still think animal fat clogs arteries, and that high cholesterol causes heart attacks.

KILLING KETO

Another casualty of the Great Fat Scare was the ketogenic diet. A diet that, again, had already shown great promise in treating diseases of the brain.

I already mentioned the promising research on migraines that had been conducted in the early 20th Century. But migraine wasn't the only condition helped by a ketogenic diet.

We've long known that a ketogenic diet works wonders for epilepsy, performing far better at preventing seizures than any pharmaceuticals. For children with frequent, sometimes daily convulsions that medications can't touch, the impact of a ketogenic diet is life-altering.

Yet, despite knowing it to be the most powerful tool in the anti-epilepsy arsenal, for nearly a century it was rarely used. And after the early 20th Century, research on the ketogenic diet ground to a halt. Why? Because of Fat Phobia. Because of misplaced fears about dietary fat.

We cast out a treatment that could transform the life of a child with unrelenting seizures or a mother with incapacitating migraines, tragically replacing it with an arsenal of less effective and more dangerous pharmaceuticals.

As mentioned, the Fat Phobia generated by The Great Fat Scare still lingers. Decades of indoctrination take time to unravel, especially amongst the generations who grew up with it as dogma. We've come quite a long way, with the popularity and widespread acceptance of the ketogenic diet (even amongst many heart doctors!) being perhaps the single best indicator of the progress we've made in undoing the damage.

Yes, the keto craze may be the most promising sign of all that The Great Fat Scare is on its last legs.

TRUST NO ONE?

It's easy to become cynical after reading a story like this. In the area of health and nutrition, it seems the "experts" are telling you one thing today, and the opposite thing tomorrow. How are you supposed to believe anything?

But, it's important to point out here that The Great Fat Scare isn't an indictment of science itself. Instead, it's a cautionary tale of what happens when we bypass the usual safeguards of science, and when we allow aggressive and unrestricted corporate influence to pervert the search for knowledge and truth.

Here we had a hunch that bypassed the usual validation process, accepted as truth before it was ever tested. Then the full weight of a government and an entire industry was thrown behind disseminating and promoting that hunch. That's *not* how things should work.

Make no mistake, we've made unbelievable progress thanks to science done the *right* way. That progress includes our willingness to identify and correct bad ideas in the face of evidence that refutes them, even if it damages the reputations of prominent scientists or a company's bottom line.

We are living amid that correction right now when it comes to our ideas about the healthfulness of dietary fat. We've seen this movie before, as the history of medical science is littered with practices once thought beneficial (bloodletting, trepanation, lobotomies, etc.) that are now the stuff of nightmares.

These corrections don't happen overnight, but ultimately the truth prevails. It's only a matter of time before Fat Phobia is eradicated from the minds of humans forever, and we'll one day look back with dismay at how we could've ever thought such a thing.

SO WHAT *WILL* HAPPEN TO MY CHOLESTEROL?

As I said, we've come a long way in the past decade or so, correcting for the major mistakes that were made in nutritional science.

But, the residue of that mistake remains. Understandably, you still may worry about the impact of more fat and cholesterol in your diet. You might still have lingering fears over saturated fat in particular, long the falsely accused villain for heart disease (the term "heart disease" is usually used to refer to atherosclerotic cardiovascular disease, or the hardening of the arteries that leads to both heart attacks and strokes).

And you will almost *certainly* encounter friends, family, and even medical professionals who harbor those fears.

These days, there are innumerable ways to refute the claim that dietary fat causes heart disease. Exploring each of those is well beyond the scope and intent of this book.

Perhaps the most convincing way is just to look at how a ketogenic diet impacts the very measures which are widely acknowledged as being markers of our risk of heart disease. You are probably familiar with the blood cholesterol test, or "lipid panel." It is also referred to as a "cardiovascular risk panel," indicating that the primary purpose of this test is to assess our risk of cardiovascular disease (including heart attacks and strokes).

The lipid panel is the test that tells you the amounts of "bad" and "good" cholesterol that are floating around in your bloodstream (outdated and misleading terms, but ones still widely used).

The lipid panel typically measures four things: 1) Total Cholesterol 2) High-density Lipiprotein Cholesterol ("HDL") 3) Low-density Lipoprotein Cholesterol ("LDL"), and 4) Triglycerides.

Recent studies have shown that total cholesterol isn't a useful predictor of heart disease. However, there is a positive correlation between total cholesterol and the risk of death. In other words, the science shows that it is much more dangerous to have a low level of cholesterol than a high one. A study published in 2019 of over 12 million adults revealed that **having a total cholesterol between 210 and 249 was associated with the lowest risk of death.**

Yet, for decades, we've been told that a total cholesterol over 200 was too high (and often placed on medication to bring it down). Why? I think you know by now.

So if your total cholesterol isn't much use for predicting your risk of heart disease, is there anything else in the lipid panel that is?

Yes.

Recent research indicates that the single best predictor of "cardiovascular risk" on the standard lipid panel (remember, the entire reason for getting this test is to assess our risk of cardiovascular disease) is the ratio of Triglycerides (TGs) to High Density Lipoprotein. Based on the latest research, I consider this ratio to be the most useful number on a standard blood cholesterol test.

Once again, TGs / HDL = the best predictor of cardiovascular disease risk.

The higher this ratio, the higher your risk of heart disease. The lower the ratio, the lower the risk. A ratio over four is associated with a high risk of heart disease. A ratio less than two is associated with a low risk, and is the ideal.

Additionally, and not coincidentally, this ratio is also an excellent predictor of whether you have large, fluffy LDL particles, or small, dense LDL particles. In the early days of cholesterol research, researchers thought *all* LDL cholesterol was bad.

We now know this isn't true. LDL particles come in different forms, varying from "large and fluffy" to "small and dense." And which kind you have makes a big difference.

The large and fluffy ones are considered benign. The small kand dense ones, on the other hand, are the ones that are found inside of artery clogging plaques. As you'd expect, then, a high ratio predicts that you have lots of small and dense particles. A low ratio predicts you have mainly large and fluffy ones.

An increase in triglycerides or a decrease in HDL will cause the ratio to go up, which increases our risk.

A decrease in triglycerides or an increase in HDL will cause the ratio to go down, which decreases our risk.

So, guess what typically happens to those two numbers when someone eats according to the Keto for Migraine plan?

Triglycerides go down (often by a lot), and HDL goes up. **And the ratio goes down.**

The very markers that the latest research shows to be the best blood indicators of cardiovascular risk *improve* on a ketogenic diet. Even the most fat-phobic cardiologist has nothing left to stand on in the face of results like this. Because the only possible explanations for those observations is that either saturated fat isn't bad for you and should not be feared or that the lipid panel is not an accurate measure of your cardiovascular risk.

You simply can't have it both ways.

One reason why we've gone off the rails here is that those who were in the business of conducting research and issuing the recommendations about what people should eat were not the ones in the clinic treating real live patients. They weren't the ones seeing people's health metrics worsen on low-fat diets.

They weren't the ones seeing that patients who ate fewer carbs and increased their consumption of good fats had better cholesterol numbers. They weren't the ones seeing, time and again, the life-changing impact that a low-to-moderate carbohydrate ancestral diet has on people's lives. They weren't the ones who, day in and day out, were confronted with clear evidence that we were wrong about the evils of dietary fat.

Those of us whose responsibility it is to do what's best for our patients didn't have the luxury of waiting around for the conventional wisdom to catch up to what we could clearly see with our own eyes. And we couldn't in good conscience continue giving advice we knew to be harmful to our patients.

It's worth pointing out here that, not only does the TGs to HDL ratio typically improve, it often drops to below one. Better yet, it drops to numbers I rarely see amongst the "typical" patient in the hospital or clinic - including those who are eating a "heart-healthy" low-fat diet under the advice of a cardiologist or nutritionist who is still unfamiliar with the latest research.

One reason I mention this is because it's common for people on a ketogenic diet to calculate this ratio, find that it's less than one, and then worry that they did it wrong.

As a physician who's been digging into this research for a decade now, and who cares about the long term health of my vital organs - especially my brain - I can say **I have zero concerns over the amount of saturated fat in my diet.**

And **I have zero concerns over the amount of saturated fat in the diet of my family members** (now that assumes they're eating a low-to-moderate carbohydrate diet - saturated fat may well be a problem for those still eating the high-carb Western diet).

The fact is that we humans have been eating significant amounts of saturated fat for millions of years. Fears about it harming us are about as misplaced as worrying that drinking water or breathing air will kill us.

WHY HASN'T MY DOCTOR TOLD ME ABOUT THIS?

Fat Phobia isn't the only obstacle standing in the way of widespread use of the ketogenic diet as a therapeutic tool for migraines and other neurological disorders.

I imagine most people think that, when they go see their doctor with a particular problem, he or she considers every possible treatment option and then selects the best one. That's exactly what I thought when I entered medical school.

Not so.

The reality is that doctors only choose from a tiny fraction of the available options. How many times have you left a doctor's office without a prescription? If it's anything but a routine physical, that's what we expect to happen.

For doctors, **the primary purpose of most office visits isn't to choose the best treatments out of all the possible treatment options, it's to select the best drug out of all the possible drug options**.

That means you aren't prescribed a drug because a drug is the best of all possible treatment options. You're prescribed a drug because, the way medicine is practiced in this day and age, this is the primary tool we have. Doctors in *medical* specialties choose from the available *medications*, and doctors in *surgical* specialties choose from the available *surgeries*.

To better understand this situation, imagine you're asked to build the best possible shelter you can, but the only materials you can use are popsicle sticks, glue, and rubber bands. You could probably make some semblance of a shelter with those materials.

And surely there are some versions of a house made of popsicle sticks, glue, and rubber bands that are better than others.

But would any of them compare to a shelter made of wood? Or bricks?

Of course not.

In medicine, we also have a very limited set of "materials" from which to choose. Even worse, like our popsicle sticks, glue, and rubber bands, our materials are poorly suited for the job at hand.

Since writing *The Migraine Miracle*, I've heard from scores of readers who, after no longer suffering from chronic migraines after decades, including going through every available prescription medication, are bewildered, at times angered, that their doctor never told them that better treatments were out there. Or they wonder how it could be that something that works so much better than prescription migraine medications hasn't become the standard treatment in every clinic around the world.

As Julia said in her Migraine Miracle Moment podcast interview, "if this were a medical device or a pharmaceutical, it would be all over the New York Times."

I've also heard from those who, upon first encountering the plan, say, "well if it worked, my doctor would've told me about it by now."

But it's important to recognize that selecting a drug to prescribe is the job! Going to a doctor and expecting a treatment beyond a prescription is like going to a podiatrist and expecting them to give you a pedicure, or going to a Chinese restaurant and expecting a pepperoni pizza. It's not what they do.

I'm not saying that's the way it *should* be in medicine, I'm saying that this is the way it is. And it's important to understand that.

Like it or not, the system we currently have strongly reinforces "drugs and surgery" as the exclusive options.

Furthermore, there are **a few additional obstacles that stand in the way of nutritional therapies like the ketogenic diet ever being incorporated into mainstream medicine's treatment ar-**

senal:

REASON #1:There's no money to be made on them.

Drugs can be patented, and they can be produced in mass quantities. Humira, the top-selling drug of 2018, made 20 billion dollars that year.

We've also conditioned everyone into believing that they're the best solution (for example, if you check the typical migraine patient support group - almost the entire conversation will revolve around various drug cocktails), which means lots of potential customers! Pills are easy money.

REASON #2: Blinded clinical trials for nutritional therapies are challenging, if not impossible, to perform. And they're expensive.

At this point in time, the randomized, double-blinded clinical trial is virtually the only way to validate a new treatment. For any new treatment to be recommended as a standard of care, it must go through this process.

But studies for nutritional therapies are hard to do and expensive. Who's going to shell out that kind of time and expense if there's no money to be made from it?

Right now, the only kind of treatment that can be tested easily in clinical trials are pharmaceuticals. We've set up the system so that the only type of treatments that even have a chance of clearing the hurdles we've required new treatments to clear are pharmaceuticals.

Coincidence?

REASON #3: Drug companies do not want people pursuing nutritional therapies (or any therapy other than a drug).

Doctors are paid very well to promote pharmaceuticals, to hype their benefits, and to denounce or suppress any alternatives. And they are often directly or indirectly encouraged to prescribe them by drug sales representatives. This all makes perfect sense - if another treatment is cheaper, safer, and better, that's bad news for their bottom line!

These payments from drug companies to doctors used to be hidden. Nowadays, companies are required to report any payments made to physicians, which was part of the Physician Payments Sunshine Act that was passed in 2010. And this information is available to the public.

So, if you hear a doctor singing the praises of a drug, and you want to know if they're being paid to do so, you can search their name in ProPublica's "Dollars for Docs" website (a Google search for "dollars for docs" will find it). You might be surprised by what you find!

Remember that Big Pharma is big business. That's where the "big" comes from!

REASON #4: Nutritional therapies are hard for doctors to use.

Doctors have an average of 7 minutes to spend with their patients these days, and that number will likely continue to shrink over time. That's nowhere near enough time to review the ins and outs of the ketogenic diet.

It is enough time, however, to write a prescription. In fact, it's essentially impossible to implement any treatment other than a pharmaceutical. One more way that the we've designed our health care system so that drugs are the only viable option to choose from.

Don't get me wrong. Medicines do have a role. And we should continue to research new drug treatments.

My point is that our view of treatments has been grossly distorted, causing us to overlook the most powerful tools we have at our disposal. Instead, we've focused exclusively on ones that are comparatively weak, often risky, under the false perception that they are the best available option, or that no other options exist.

KEYS FROM CHAPTER 2:

1) Despite the promise it showed in treating neurological conditions, including migraine, clinicians and researchers abandoned the ketogenic diet for nearly a century over concerns about dietary fat.

2) This fear of fat, aka the "Great Fat Scare," was entirely misplaced, and is now a cautionary tale about how egos and corporate interests can distort science.

3) You can prove the dietary fat and heart disease hypothesis wrong yourself, as other ketogenic dieters have done. The typical response to the *Keto for Migraine* diet is for the ratio of Triglycerides to HDL to go down, often considerably. Research indicates this ratio is the best predictor of heart dis-

ease risk.

4) There are multiple reasons why nutritional therapies like the ketogenic diet are not typically considered as treatment options in Western medicine, none of which have anything to do with its effectiveness. For several reasons, pharmaceuticals are the primary treatment option doctors have, so they are unlikely to be aware of or recommend alternatives, even if they are more effective.

CHAPTER 3: KETO EXPLAINED

WHAT YOU'LL LEARN IN THIS CHAPTER: *In this chapter, you'll learn what happens inside the body on a ketogenic diet, how ketone bodies are made, and reasons why ketones may be especially beneficial to the migraine brain.*

It's about time we discussed precisely what "keto" is! As I mentioned in the introduction, keto has recently hit escape velocity in popular culture. It's become so ubiquitous, so woven into the fabric of the world around us, that it's easy to only have a superficial understanding of it. Like a word we've used all our lives but have never stopped to ask where it originated.

Given the way it's so often portrayed these days, it's also easy to think that "keto" is just a name for one of a gajillion diet plans, like "Jenny Craig," or "Weight Watchers." Like other diets, you may expect that it's ultimately destined for the graveyard of fad diets, killed off by the next latest and greatest craze.

But keto is different. And it isn't going anywhere. Why am I so confident that it will beat the odds?

For starters, *because it works.*

It works really well for weight loss, and a host of other things. Results always speak for themselves. Its viral growth hasn't been driven by deceptive marketing, but by word of mouth. By friends telling friends "you *have* to try this."

Furthermore, it's grounded in solid science. And the only reason it's just now coming into its own is that Fat Phobia had kept it locked away for so long. Now that the truth about fat is out, it has cleared the way for keto to take its rightful place as a powerful and versatile nutritional therapy.

Rather than being the pithy name for the latest fad diet, "keto" instead refers to a physiological process known as nutritional ketosis. And while it isn't necessary whatsoever to know all the precise details of the relevant biochemistry, it is quite useful to have a basic grasp of what's happening inside the body when we're in ketosis.

As I said before, having some basic knowledge and understanding about the underlying principles of what we're doing, rather than memorizing a set of rules about what to eat, is key to long term success.

KETONE BODY MAGIC

Imagine if tomorrow a new drug was unveiled that did the following:

- **Improved your mental clarity,** or your ability to think clearly, and overall eliminated your dreaded "brain fog."

- **Improved your focus and attention**, sharpening your mind so that you could easily focus on one task for extended periods, immune to the omnipresent distractions of modern life.

- **Curbed your appetite**, allowing you to lose weight without starving yourself, or feeling deprived.

- **Helped the brain to run more efficiently** so that it produced less of the toxic metabolic waste that's been strongly linked to neurodegenerative disorders like Alzheimer's and Parkinson's.

- **Calmed overactive brain cells,** or areas of "hyper-excitability," such that it lowered anxiety, promoted calmness and serenity, and reduced the likelihood of seizures and migraines.

- **Starved and killed pre-cancerous cells** in your body, making it impossible for them to grow into cancer cells.

- **Was as safe or safer than any other drug on the market**.

Again, imagine a pharmaceutical that could do all of those things. It's the stuff of dreams for drug companies.

Needless to say, if a drug like this were indeed to hit the market tomorrow, it would be a blockbuster.

Now, what if I told you that your body can make this drug all by itself? For free!

Nice to meet you, ketones.

So, perhaps you now understand why I say that "keto" is here to stay. Your next question I'm sure is "how do I get my body to manufacture this magical molecule?"

HOW TO MAKE A KETONE

Every living thing requires energy to stay alive. The ability to produce energy is the signature difference between a living and a dead thing. We generate that energy by burning fuel.

From this perspective, the body is no different than a car engine. Both extract the energy inside of fuel by burning it.

One of the more unique features of human biology is that our bodies can run on more than one fuel source. This flexibility in how we generate energy is part of what has allowed our species to survive in such a wide range of habitats.

One of those fuel sources that we can burn for energy is glucose, which is a kind of sugar. "Sugars" are a group of molecules that share similar chemical structures and behaviors. But, when we talk of "blood sugar," what we're actually referring to is our blood glucose.

Sometimes that glucose in our blood comes directly from the food we eat. Other times it comes from breaking down a complex sugar that we store, known as glycogen.

However, the amount of sugar our body can store is small. We can only provide a small amount of energy by draining our body's sugar reservoirs, around 400 calories. That's well under half the number of calories that a typical person needs in one day just to fuel basic life-supporting functions.

The other fuel we can burn for energy is fat. Or, to use the more technical term, fatty acids.

As it is with sugar, the fat we use for energy can come from the food that we eat, or it can come from the fat that we store in our fat tissues. And we humans are great at storing fat. A 50-year-old woman of average height and healthy body fat has 120 - 150,000 calories stored in her fat tissue.

That's enough calories to meet her energy needs for two months!

Now, at any given moment in our day, we're burning a mix of glucose and fat for energy. The relative proportion that we're burning at any given moment depends on many factors. We can influence those relative amounts through what we eat by adjusting the amount of carbohydrates and fat in our meals.

Once we hit a certain level of fat burning, it fills up our fat burning machinery in the liver. In technical terms, our liver's first fat burning pathway becomes "saturated." Like an assembly line, there's a limit to how fast that machinery can work. When we exceed that limit, fat gets re-routed into another pathway that converts it into ketone bodies.

So, for our purposes here, the basic thing to remember is that ketones are made from fats that are absorbed (from the stomach) or released (from the fat tissue) into the bloodstream, but only *after* the first fat-burning pathway in the liver has reached its maximum capacity. This is why it takes a certain amount of fat in the bloodstream to produce ketone bodies.

Now you understand how ketones get made in the liver. But what happens next? Why does the liver make these things in the first place, and what role do they play in the body?

Ketones serve as another form of fuel for the body; however, only certain tissues can convert ketones into energy. As we've reviewed, the liver makes our ketones; but, liver cells are actually unable to use those ketones for energy.

Instead, the ketones made in the liver are released into the blood, where they then travel to other organs that *can* use them for fuel, including the muscles, kidneys, heart and, most importantly for our purposes, the brain.

One of the unique features of the brain is that, unlike almost all of the other tissues, it can't burn fat for fuel. So, when there's not a lot of glucose around, the brain's only alternative is ketones.

On the standard, high-carb Western diet, the brain is burning sugar as its primary source of fuel virtually all of the time. The damage caused by our brain burning sugar all the time appears to be tremendous, as that damage is linked to all manner of neurological problems, including migraine.

On a ketogenic diet, the brain is instead burning ketones as its main source of fuel.

CLEAN ENERGY FOR YOUR BRAIN

To understand how burning ketones benefits our brain, I'm going to first take a brief detour into the topic of energy. I promise it'll all make sense in the end, and give you a better understanding of why so many people who care about improving brain health and function are so excited about ketones.

These days, the world is becoming increasingly concerned about the kind of fuels we use to generate the energy that powers all the many technologies that we now rely on as part of modern life.

Why? Well, there are really two things we care about most. When it comes to generating energy, the first is how much energy we can get from a given amount of fuel. All things being equal, the more energy we can produce for a given amount of fuel, the less time and resources we have to devote to obtaining fuel.

The ideal fuel provides a lot of energy for a small amount of stuff. We can get more with less effort.

The second thing we care about is how much waste we generate when we burn fuel. The smoke of a wood-burning fire contains far more pollutants than the smoke of a propane-burning fire, which we can see clearly with our own eyes. More waste means more mess to clean up, as anyone who's cooked with a charcoal and a gas-burning grill can attest!

And the more mess, the higher the chances that those waste by-products will cause trouble. As you probably know, one of the waste products of burning fossil fuels is carbon dioxide, which, when added to the atmosphere, traps heat and contributes to rising global temperatures. For this reason, finding fuels that burn cleaner has become a pressing concern for us all.

In sum, **the ideal fuel gives a lot of energy in a small package and generates a minimal amount of waste.**

What's this have to do with ketones, you ask? Well, as I've already discussed, our body also burns fuel for energy, in the form of glucose, fatty acids, and ketones - with the brain only able to burn glucose and ketones.

It turns out that when we compare ketones to glucose on these two major characteristics of concern, ketones win on both accounts.

First, **ketones provide more energy for the same amount of stuff as glucose.**

Second, **ketones generate less waste than glucose.** By quite a bit, it seems.

This fact about ketones already seems pretty good on face value. But these two advantages of ketones over glucose may hold tremendous promise for preventing the most feared diseases of the brain.

Just like carbon dioxide in the atmosphere, or the build up of ash in your charcoal grill, an overabundance of waste gums up the works. Our bodies and brains do have their own waste removal resources, but they can only do so much. All it takes is for us to create more waste than we remove for things to start breaking down.

And what is a signature feature of the most common neuro-degenerative conditions like Alzheimer's, Lewy Body Dementia, and Parkinson's? Too much waste.

The fact that burning ketones produces less waste than burning glucose is precisely why keto is now viewed by many in this field as an area of tremendous promise, and why the standard high-carb, high-waste-producing Western diet is thought by many to be a key factor in the development of these diseases.

It's also why, in my opinion, anyone who cares about the health of their brain (which should mean every single person) should integrate keto into their lives in some way, shape, or form. It's entirely possible that adopting such a strategy can keep conditions like Alzheimer's from ever developing, even amongst those who are genetically vulnerable.

The fact that ketones burn cleaner also may explain, at least in part, why a ketogenic diet can be such a powerful weapon against migraines.

KETONES - DEFENDERS OF OXIDATIVE DAMAGE

There is much we still don't know about migraines, especially when it comes to what is happening down at the level of cellular interactions, or the level of molecules. Though that's not to say we haven't made considerable progress.

One theory about how migraines develop that's been gaining support is that migraines are a response to oxidative stress. I imagine you may have heard the term oxidative stress before but might not have a clear understanding of what it means.

Normal metabolism, which is the process of extracting energy from food, generates reactive oxygen species (ROS). Like hammer-wielding vandals smashing anything in sight, these unstable molecules can wreak havoc if left unchecked, damaging cell membranes, proteins, and our DNA. Research indicates that this damage is likely a driving factor in many diseases, as well as a key factor in the aging process.

So, the sooner we can eradicate these biochemical vandals after they're produced, the less damage they cause. And we have proteins in our body, known as "anti-oxidants," whose job it is to do precisely that.

To review, reactive oxygen species are generated in the course of normal metabolism. These guys can wreak havoc in the body, so we have various anti-oxidants that try to remove them as fast as possible.

If the amount of ROS's produced exceeds what our anti-oxidants can remove, then we are said to be under "oxidative stress."

As mentioned, recent evidence indicates that those who suffer from migraines have a higher level of oxidative stress. And a theory has been proposed that migraines are a response to oxidative stress, or that migraines occur when our systems for eradicating reactive oxygen species have been overwhelmed.

While there are many potential explanations why ketogenic diets help prevent migraines - and it's entirely likely that there is more than one reason - here we have a theory of the origin of migraines that would predict a ketogenic diet to be beneficial.

Why is that? Remember that ketones burn cleaner, meaning fewer waste products are produced when we metabolize them for energy. That includes fewer reactive oxygen species, or free radicals. **A ketogenic diet produces less waste, and increases the number of anti-oxidants, both of which contribute to a reduction in oxidative stress.**

So, if migraines are a response to oxidative stress, then eating in a way that reduces oxidative stress would mean fewer migraines, which is what we see happening to migraineurs in ketosis!

Furthermore, since oxidative stress is linked to aging, cancer, and a host of other diseases, being in ketosis also means slower aging, and a reduced risk of all manner of conditions.

Now, all that being said, we needn't know *why* keto works to use it. And it may be quite some time before we have those answers. But nobody needs to wait until we have all the answers.

It'd be one thing if nutritional ketosis carried significant risks. But that's not the case. **Ketosis is a natural physiologic state, one that humans have had experience with for millions of years.** Thanks to the seasonal availability and scarcity of carbohydrates, it was a physiologic state our ancestors likely spent considerable time in.

The average person today, on the other hand, spends much less time than our ancestors would have in ketosis. This relative absence of nutritional ketosis is one of many possible explanations for why migraines, like other chronic conditions such as diabetes, heart disease, cancer, and dementia, are diseases of civilization, only occurring when human brains are subjected to our evolutionarily novel, modern environment.

KEYS FROM CHAPTER 3:

1) When ketones are produced, the brain can use them for energy in place of glucose.

2) Ketones generate less waste than glucose, a primary reason why ketosis is considered a protective strategy against neurodegenerative diseases (Alz-

heimer's, Parkinson's, etc.), and may be one of the reasons why it protects against migraines.

3) Ketones help to reduce and defend against oxidative stress. Oxidative stress has been linked to the generation of migraines.

4) Nutritional ketosis is a normal physiological state and one that our ancestors spent much of their time in for millions of years.

5) If a drug could do all the things that keto could do, it'd be considered the magic pill everyone wishes would exist.

CHAPTER 4 - THE KETO FOR MIGRAINE PLAN

WHAT YOU'LL LEARN IN THIS CHAPTER: *It's the moment you've been waiting for! There are many roads to keto. Some may lead you straight to The Beast. Others can be one of your most powerful weapons against him. In this chapter, we'll review the basic principles of the Keto for Migraine plan, designed to maximize the Beast-slaying benefits of keto.*

Laura is a 50-year-old woman whose migraines began at age 12. Until she reached her late 20s, her migraines were occasional, occurring maybe once per month. She saw her first neurologist at age 28 and was given a prescription for sumatriptan.

Over the next two decades, her migraines steadily escalated, coming more often and with greater intensity. Over that time, she was placed on a veritable smorgasbord of medications. They included amitriptyline, topiramate, propranolol, and she had cycled through virtually every triptan on the market.

She now takes oral zolmitriptan when she has an attack, though she doesn't use it more than twice a week as instructed by her neurologist. She no longer uses over-the-counter medications, as they do nothing.

She's also tried Botox, acupuncture, chiropractic, and massage. She's been to the Emergency Department on numerous occasions for migraine attacks that wouldn't abate after several days.

While perusing a Facebook migraine group one day, she comes across a post from someone sharing their successes with a ketogenic diet. "After twenty years of nothing working, finally something that does!" the post says and goes on to encourage other migraineurs to give keto a try.

Excited, and with little to lose, Laura begins researching the keto diet. She's heard of some friends who've been using it to lose weight, but until this point didn't know it could help with her migraines.

She begins looking up "keto recipes" on Google and Pinterest. She buys a book on keto from Amazon. She joins a few keto-related Facebook groups. After a few days with her information-gathering phase complete, she takes the plunge and goes keto.

The first ten days are challenging, which she expected. Her research had prepared her to experience symptoms like these as her body made the transition into ketosis. Her energy is lower than usual. A dull, diffuse headache develops. It's less intense than her typical migraines, but present most of the time. She presses on, though, and the symptoms dissipate, as she'd been told they would.

She continues her keto experiment for six more weeks. Over that time, she loses 6 pounds, which she's pleased about. That dip in her energy is gone. If anything, she feels more energetic than she has in many years.

But her migraines are no better. In fact, according to her headache diary, they're *worse*.

Though the weight loss and extra energy are nice, she decides that's not worth more visits from The Beast. So, she stops eating keto.

She returns to that original Facebook post that prompted her to go keto in the first place and comments, "I tried it, and unfortunately, it didn't work for me. I think my migraines even got worse. I guess I'm one of the unlucky ones it doesn't work for."

Though her name is fictional, Laura's story is not. And it's a story that has become increasingly common as the popularity of the ketogenic diet has surged in recent years. That's a major reason why I decided to write this book, in fact.

Because Laura's experience is entirely preventable. In this chapter, you'll learn what I've learned helping thousands of migraine sufferers implement a ketogenic diet so that Laura's story doesn't become yours, too!

KETO MADNESS

Recently, I did a Google search for keto recipes. What did I find?

Well over half were for keto substitutes for high-carb treats. Keto breads, keto pies, keto ice cream, keto cinnamon rolls, keto cheesecake, chocolate fat bombs, and on and on and on.

Sigh.

As I mentioned earlier, one of the reasons for writing this book is because I know how transformative a ketogenic diet can be for the migraineur. Yet, I also know that the commercialized version of the ketogenic diet that you'll find on Pinterest boards, Facebook posts, and magazines in the checkout line of the grocery store are almost sure to make migraines worse, not better.

A ketogenic diet is any way of eating that leads to the production of ketones. That's it. And there are countless ways you could eat to achieve that. Every single person in the world could go keto tomorrow, and each person could have his or her entirely unique version.

For virtually everyone, changing to a dietary pattern that stimulates ketones will mean a significant departure from their regular eating habits. Number one, the kinds of foods will change. Chances are so will meal times, meal frequency, calories consumed per meal, and so on.

The point is that a great many variables are going to change for anyone who is adopting a ketogenic diet. This means that the addition of circulating ketones to your body and brain is only one of those variables.

The ketones themselves do great things for the brain, including doing great things for the brains of migraineurs. But what about all those other changes? We want to make sure that all of those other changes we make to stimulate ketosis **don't end up tipping the migraine scales in the wrong direction.**

Put another way, we could divide the set of all possible ketogenic diets into versions that reduce migraines, versions that have no impact, and versions that make them worse. Like all the others I've worked with, you're interested only in versions that fall in the first category.

Even if you've decided to go keto for some reason besides migraine protection, that still applies. For example, if you're a migraineur looking to reap the fat loss benefits of a ketogenic diet, the last thing you want is for it to make your migraines worse! Just not worth it.

Over the past five years, as we've held numerous 30-day

Keto Blast challenges, shepherding thousands of migraineurs through the process of going keto, we've learned so much about what works and what hurts. And over the years, we've been able to use what we've learned to optimize the ketogenic diet for migraine sufferers.

It's easy when going keto to become laser-focused on *just* producing ketones. It's easy to think that all that matters is getting into ketosis and that the path you take to get there is irrelevant.

But how you get there is *very* relevant. In fact, for the migraineur, how you get there makes all the difference in the world.

When I talked about the ketogenic diet in the book *The Migraine Miracle* back in 2013, hardly anyone knew what keto was, much less that it could be a powerful weapon against migraine. For most readers, the section on the ketogenic diet was the first time they'd even heard the term.

Then the keto craze began, and word began to spread about its migraine-busting benefits, too.

A few years ago, we started seeing stories like Laura's trickling in. Someone would hear that a ketogenic diet was helpful for migraines. They'd then begin collecting information, surfing the internet, gathering recipes from Google searches and Pinterest boards, join a "keto" Facebook group or three, and get started.

Then, after a few weeks, to their great disappointment, they'd notice their migraines were no better. Sometimes they'd gotten worse. Why? Because they hadn't taken a migraine-friendly path to keto. Moreover, they didn't even realize there was such a thing, or that the path to keto even mattered.

And yet, what did they conclude about their foray into keto? That it didn't work. That they must just be one of the unlucky ones that it doesn't help. But of course, that conclusion ignores all of the other variables that changed when they went keto and their impact on migraines.

This again speaks to the importance of a holistic approach to health, where it's never about the impact of any one thing, but rather the combined impact of all of our health behaviors.

Imagine that, after a routine physical, my doctor tells me I need to start walking three miles a day. My blood pressure, blood sugar, and weight are all creeping into the unhealthy range, and she believes this is the single best thing I could do to reverse those trends.

So, being the good patient that I am, I decide to follow her advice.

But I want something to help hold me accountable because I know that will significantly increase my chances of sticking with my new walking habit. So I look for a walking group to join.

The first group I find is a group of dog owners who meet every morning to go for a three-mile walk with their four-legged friends. That's my first option.

The second group I find is a group of twenty-somethings who meet up at midnight every night for a three-mile bar crawl, hopping from one bar to the next, so that by the end of their three-mile walk, everyone is deliriously drunk.

I decide the second group sounds like more fun, so I join up with the bar-hopping twenty-somethings, getting my recommended three-mile walk in each and every night.

A year later, I go back for another physical.

My doctor walks into the room with my lab results in her hand and a grave look on her face.

"I don't understand this. Everything has gotten worse. Your

weight and your blood pressure are way up, and your liver is severely inflamed."

"You've got to be kidding!" I exclaim. "I've been walking three miles a day just like you said to!"

Of course, this is a ridiculous scenario. And of course it would be absurd for me to think that my downturn in health was because of my new walking habit or to conclude that walking was *bad* for my health because it ignores all of those other behaviors that occurred in tandem with my new walking habit.

Sure, walking three miles a day on its own makes me healthier. But, on balance, it can't compete with the negative impact of all those other behaviors I added with it.

Likewise, if you do the pub crawl version of keto, and you don't see your desired results, it's not fair or reasonable to conclude that keto failed you, right?

Our objective with the *Keto for Migraine* diet is to ensure that all of the changes that we make in the name of keto are moving us closer to where we want to be.

Carbs, fats, and proteins - what ratios??

As I've mentioned, ketones are produced in the liver when we overwhelm the liver's fat-burning machinery, so that those excess fats are diverted to where they can be converted into ketones.

And there are really two places that those fats can come from. The first is from the food we eat. The second is from the fat that's stored in our body (remember that most of us have two or more month's worth of energy stored in our fat tissue!).

Getting fat from food is easy. We just eat it.

But reaping the full range of benefits from a ketogenic diet requires us to burn our body fat as well. And that isn't as easy, as the billions of people who've struggled year-after-year to lose weight can attest.

One of the huge problems with the standard high-carb Western diet and the reason obesity rates have skyrocketed as we've eaten more refined carbs, is that it makes it hard for us to access our stored body fat. In a sense, it's locked up, and our body isn't making the keys.

Fat doesn't just magically seep out of our fat stores whenever we need it. Instead, there's a whole set of metabolic machinery made of proteins and other molecules whose job it is to get it out of the fat tissue, carry it through the blood, and get it into the tissues that can burn it for energy.

If you're eating a diet that's high in carbohydrates, your body doesn't need that fat burning machinery. Why not? Because you're providing all of your energy through the carbs you eat.

And since so many of the carbs we eat today are purposefully made in ways that make it hard for us to stop eating them, we often end up eating more energy than we need at each meal. We store that extra energy as fat.

So on the typical high-carb Western diet, we're relying on the carbs we eat as our primary energy source, we have less use for our body's fat mobilizing machinery, and we're often shoving *extra* energy into our fat tissues each time we eat.

In other words, anyone who's been on a standard Western diet for any length of time is not good at getting fat out of their fat tissue. The apparatus needed to do so isn't around.

If we want to get the most out of keto, however, we must change that.

Fortunately, we can! And, for most, the solution is very straightforward. Ditch the carbs. Add the fat. We'll get into the specifics here in just a moment.

KETO FOR MIGRAINE - MINDING THE PILLARS

Time to recap.

Our primary goal with a ketogenic diet is to increase the amount of fat we burn for energy, past the threshold needed to produce ketones. Doing so requires eating sufficient amounts of fat in our diet, and improving our ability to mobilize and burn fat from our fat tissues (improving our "fat-burning" capacity).

There are countless ways to make that happen. **Our goal is to choose a way that's migraine friendly** so that we can reap all the Beast Slaying benefits of keto.

Let's review what we don't want to do.

Some of you may be familiar with my 3 Pillars of Migraine Protection. For those that aren't, the three pillars are the essential components required for migraine freedom. Like the support structures of a building, if any one of them is weak, then the edifice will crumble.

What are the pillars?

The FIRST PILLAR is the elimination of rebound headaches or medication-induced vulnerability. I've written and spoke extensively about this topic, so I won't go into depth here (you can find several episodes on the topic on the Migraine Miracle Moment podcast).

But here's the gist: one of the significant downsides to the medications that are taken for migraine relief - the migraine "abortives," as they're commonly known - is that they help in the short term, but hurt in the long term. They can help relieve an attack

from the Beast (though, as I'm sure you know, not a¹
they also make us more vulnerable to future attacks.

Medications vary in terms of how vulnerable they make us to
a future attack, which I've dubbed their "Future Migraine Risk
Score." This score, which ranges from 1 to 10, is based on my
professional experience using these medications, along with
the published research on rebound headaches.

On this scale, the higher the score, the greater the risk of experiencing another attack in the near future. Recently, I reviewed
the various migraine medications and created a guide to the Future Migraine Risk Score for each drug, which you can download
by going to **mymigrainemiracle.com/drugscore**.

It's important to note that this effect of the migraine medications adds up with each dose. The more we take, the more
vulnerable we become to a future migraine. So the meds cause
the frequency of our migraines to go up, which usually ends up
causing us to take more meds, which further increases the frequency of our migraines, and so on.

It's a vicious cycle, and it's incredibly common (most migraine
patients I see in my clinic for the first time are stuck in this
cycle). And it's not uncommon for people to get stuck in this
cycle for *decades*, in part because no one ever told them this
would happen.

This effect of the medications is potent and, if not addressed,
can undermine all of our other efforts to achieve migraine freedom, which is why eliminating rebound is one of the three pillars.

In the story I opened with, Laura is taking a triptan twice a
week, which she continues to do after going keto. This "twice-a-
week-or-less" rule has long been the traditional advice given by
neurologists to migraine patients to reduce the risk of rebound
headaches. Like Laura many of my fellow migraineurs have dis-

covered that this number is much too high, as it dramatically underestimates the impact of abortive medications on increasing the risk of a future migraine.

For years, I gave the same advice - limit triptans, or migraine abortives, to two days a week or less. Unknowingly, that advice was **serving as a critical impediment to people making progress towards migraine freedom**. And it was a key impediment in my own progress as well.

Personally, I won't ever take another triptan, and I now have a very high threshold for taking any medication for migraine relief. In the past, triptans were my first option. Now they are my last because the drawbacks just aren't worth it.

Now, had I not discovered a powerful strategy for preventing migraines, and had I not discovered a host of other ways to relieve a migraine attack that don't require a pill, I wouldn't be able to say that (you'll find my 11 Drug-Free Strategies for Ending A Migraine in the Supplemental Guide, which you can grab at ketoformigraine.com/guide)

There are many ways to go about minimizing or eliminating the impact of abortive migraine medications so that they don't undermine your success with a ketogenic diet. Some people flush them down the toilet and vow never to take them again. Others taper their use down over time.

The real key to success is making an informed and educated decision about how the migraine meds are used, one that fully factors in their risks. The biggest mistake we've made in the health care community is in telling people to use them as their first resort, to take something "at the first sign of a migraine." That's excellent advice if you want to create an epidemic of rebound headaches (which we've done). It's also great advice if you want to sell lots of pharmaceuticals.

The primary shift that has helped the people I work with the most is **to change from thinking of the migraine relief medications as a first option and switching to thinking of them as a last option**. That one shift in thinking will drastically reduce the chances that the drugs will sabotage your chance of success.

The SECOND PILLAR is the establishment of metabolic flexibility.

We've already discussed our ability as humans to burn multiple different substances to generate the energy that powers our body.

We can burn carbs, aka sugars. We can burn fats. And we can burn ketones.

As discussed earlier, on the standard Western diet that's high in carbohydrates, most people are burning carbs for their energy much of the time. Those carbs are coming from the foods they eat.

A diet that's high in carbs, especially the refined kind (sugar and flour, including many that are gluten free) that are so commonplace nowadays, leads to the accumulation of excess body fat. Moreover, a diet high in carbs makes it harder for us to access that excess body fat to use for fuel.

Our stores of fat become a one-way street - fat goes in but doesn't come out. Those in this situation, which probably describes most Westerners, have become metabolically *inflexible.*

Someone who is metabolically inflexible has difficulty switching between different fuel sources. These days, it's usually difficulty changing from burning carbs to burning fat. Metabolic inflexibility, which is a direct consequence of diet, is a crucial factor in obesity, and likely many of the other diseases of our time.

As mentioned in chapter 3, achieving ketosis requires that we access that body fat. In a sense, our body has to "learn" how to readily access our stored body fat again. This learning process involves building up the machinery the body uses to mobilize and burn fat, which requires turning on the genes that code for that machinery. That means during ketosis, we're making changes all the way down to the level of our DNA. Cool stuff, right?!

Now, what do you think life is like for someone who is metabolically inflexible, who is only really able to derive the energy they need from the carbs they eat?

They'd experience a lot of ups and downs in their energy levels, right? After a meal, they get a burst of energy. Since carbs are absorbed and metabolized pretty quickly, that energy would dissipate rapidly. So, a little while after that last meal, energy levels crash, and ravenous hunger ensues.

So, someone who is metabolically inflexible and dependent on carbs will have lots of ups and downs in energy (and mood!) throughout the day, and will usually require snacks in between meals to compensate. These ups and downs in energy also trigger major fluctuations in hormone levels throughout the day.

Since major fluctuations in energy and hormones are a primary driver of migraines, **metabolic inflexibility will also mean many more visits from the Beast.**

By contrast, someone who is metabolically *flexible* can burn energy from the food they eat, as well as from the fat in their fat stores. So, what is life like for someone who is metabolically flexible, and who can easily tap into their ample stores of body fat to meet their energy needs?

Quite wonderful!

No longer dependent on eating a meal, someone who is metabolically flexible can go extended time between eating without any dips in energy level or mood. And gone is the roller coaster of energy and hormones that are familiar to so many of us.

With those migraine-provoking fluctuations in energy levels and hormones now out of the picture, metabolic flexibility also means many fewer visits from the Beast.

As discussed, becoming metabolically flexible is a process, and one that doesn't happen overnight. The body must make significant changes, all the way down to the level of DNA as we "learn" how to be metabolically flexible (or more accurately, "relearn," as this should be the normal state of human physiology).

But, this transition to metabolic flexibility is often *experienced* as a sudden surge in energy levels, along with the welcome disappearance of the cycles of hunger in between meals that most people had accepted as a fact of life.

And it's also often accompanied by a significant reduction in migraines, as we'd expect. This is why restoring the body to its natural state of metabolic flexibility is one of our 3 Pillars of Protection for migraine freedom. The metabolic inflexibility caused by the standard high-carb Western diet fuels the Beast, and makes a life with migraines a virtual certainty.

So, what can you do to restore your ability to burn body fat for energy? Stop eating what caused you to lose that ability in the first place!

The primary way we restore our ability to burn stored body fat for energy is by reducing the amount of carbohydrates in the diet, especially the processed and refined kind. A big reason why low carb and ketogenic diets have become such popular weight loss tools is because, by restoring the body's natural fat-burning capabilities, they allow us to burn body fat without feeling hungry all the time (you *can* lose weight on a high-carb diet, but it requires always feeling hungry and miserable, which is why the long-term success rate is so dismal).

Since achieving nutritional ketosis requires that we eat a minimal amount of carbohydrates, it is a potent stimulator of metabolic flexibility. And this is likely a significant reason why it's become such a powerful weapon against migraines as well.

Now, as I said, we can achieve nutritional ketosis, and promote metabolic flexibility, by merely dropping carbs in the diet.

But, as I've already discussed at length, that alone doesn't guarantee protection against migraines, as it's possible to do so and still make our migraines worse. The key to *not* doing so is minding our 3rd Pillar.

The THIRD PILLAR is the elimination of mismatch foods and behaviors.

Every single species of animal on planet earth has its own set of foods and environmental conditions that it needs to thrive. In other words, every animal has a natural habitat.

Panda bears can't live in the same places or eat the same things as wolves. Nor can kangaroos and clownfish.

And the particular kinds of foods and environments that every animal is best adapted to is determined by that animal's evolutionary history. Animals are most likely to thrive in the habitats their species has been living in the longest.

We all know this to be true. We all know that each animal has a unique set of foods that it needs to thrive. We apply this principle to the care of our pets every day.

And yet, by and large, we've forgotten to apply this same principle to ourselves.

But of course, we humans are no different. We are also best adapted to a particular set of foods and environmental conditions or habitats. In those habitats, we thrive. When we escape the human habitat, when our lives are mismatched to that of our ancestors, we get sick.

Just like any other animal.

Moreover, most of the chronic health conditions doctors like myself see these days are driven by this mismatch. Mismatch diseases are so prevalent now because the habitat we humans find ourselves in has changed so much in such a short period.

For over 2 million years, the habitats that our human ancestors lived in were more or less the same. Life for a human 20,000 years ago looked pretty much as it did for one 200,000 years ago. In both cases, we were hunter-gatherers living in the wild.

The first big shift came when we transitioned from hunting and gathering to farming as our means of acquiring food. And our habitat shift accelerated dramatically during the industrial age when we began making food in factories. Yet, our body and brain remain finely tuned to the life and foods of the wild hunting-and-gathering human.

Just as a wolf would fall ill on a diet of bamboo and a panda on one of elk meat, so to do we when we eat food that's not part of our natural diet. And we are now in the midst of a massive public health crisis because we've overlooked this basic biological principle.

As Dan Lieberman, chair of the Department of Evolutionary Biology at Harvard University, states, "I don't think it is possible to overemphasize just how important mismatch diseases are." I couldn't agree more.

But there's good news. Knowing that mismatch is the driver of chronic disease provides us a roadmap for what to do about it. When we treat these conditions by reducing that mismatch, we can achieve results far surpassing what modern medicines have to offer. Modern medicines are band-aids, while efforts to reduce mismatch address root causes.

Migraines are a mismatch disease occurring when our brain is faced with the demands of living in a world well outside the bounds of our evolutionary experience, of living in the wrong habitat.

A big part of that habitat mismatch comes from the foods that we eat. For one, the diet of our ancestors was significantly lower in carbohydrates. And refined carbohydrates, which now form the bulk of calories the typical westerner eats, weren't available at all.

Meat was eaten year-round, along with root vegetables and fruits when in season (though the fruits that were eaten then had nowhere near the sugar content of those we find in the grocery store, as we've bred many fruits over thousands of generations to increase their sugar content). Establishing the second pillar of metabolic flexibility takes care of the carbohydrate mismatch since you cannot become metabolically flexible without removing processed carbs from the diet.

When it comes to food, the concept is simple: stop eating foods your body is poorly equipped to process and digest, and that cause us harm when we eat them. This includes:

- Foods with substances that impair digestion or damage our gut lining (e.g., plant lectins, which are found abundantly in grains).

- Foods that have been engineered (and usually made in factories) to hijack the brain so that we eat more than we need (e.g., packaged convenience foods).

- Foods with substances that trigger an immune response (particularly in the setting of a damaged gut lining), leading to systemic inflammation and likely compromising the blood-brain barrier, the wall that protects the brain from harmful substances in the blood.

The problem with the version of the ketogenic diet most people eat these days, and the reason it can easily lead to migraines getting worse, is that it is often still mismatched. While lower in carbohydrates, **it is still not a diet that's appropriate for a human.**

In terms of the 3 Pillars of Migraine Protection, **the typical ketogenic diet may strengthen Pillar 2 while at the same time weakening Pillar 3**.

So a migraine-friendly ketogenic diet is simply one that only includes human food. The great tragedy of our time is that so few know what that means!

Now, why is it that many people can get by eating a ketogenic diet that includes non-human food without any apparent problems? Because while the typical person eating non-human food suffers by developing a chronic illness over several years, migraineurs suffer by experiencing throbbing, unbearable head pain in a matter of hours. For the non-migraineur, the consequences just aren't as immediate.

What does a ketogenic diet that's appropriate for a human look like? Here are the guidelines:

THE KETO FOR MIGRAINE GUIDELINES

1) Eat animal and low-carb plant foods.

Humans are well adapted to eating every kind of animal, whether they live on land or sea. And animal foods are the most nutrient-dense foods we can eat.

Meat (beef, lamb, and bison are ideal, along with chicken and seafood) and non-starchy vegetables (arugula, kale, spinach, Brussels sprout, chard, broccoli, green beans, collards, celery, green and red peppers) should comprise most of the diet.

2) Avoid foods with flour and added sugar.

Tragically, flour and sugar (both refined carbohydrates) are the primary source of calories for most westerners these days. Just by eliminating these from the diet (neither of which are appropriate food for humans) and replacing them with something else will drastically reduce your daily carb intake, moving you on the road to migraine freedom.

3) Cook with butter, ghee (clarified butter), animal fat (lard, tallow, duck fat), coconut oil, olive oil, or avocado oil

One of the central problems with our modern diet is the enormous increase in our consumption of vegetable and seed oils, which is likely a key driver of chronic diseases. These are oils that can only be made in factories with industrial-age machinery, and so would've been impossible for our ancestors to have consumed.

Because they are cheap and easy to make, and because for a while we made the drastic mistake of thinking they were healthier than animal fat, they've made their way into virtually every packaged convenience food. The good news here is that healthy fats taste much better.

4) Limit dairy to butter, ghee, heavy cream, and soft and un-aged cheeses (mozzarella, ricotta, goat, mascarpone).

This recommendation comes from our direct experience in working with thousands of migraineurs implementing a ketogenic diet. I've covered the complexities of dairy elsewhere, so I won't go into that here. The bottom line is that dairy can be problematic for those who don't have robust gut health. Given that migraines are likely an indicator of impaired gut function, it's reasonable to avoid foods that can be problematic in that setting. Like dairy. Or, more specifically, dairy protein. Better safe than sorry.

The upside here is that, by following the Migraine Miracle plan, you'll be healing your gut each and every day. We've worked with many folks who have successfully reintroduced other forms of dairy after being on the plan for a while (and who've reached Phase 4 on the Timeline of Migraine Freedom), presumably because, by eating only human food, they've restored their gut health.

5) Aim for 4 hours between the last meal of the day and bedtime.

One of the glorious benefits of achieving metabolic flexibility is that it becomes much easier to go for extended times between meals. Again, we're not supposed to feel hungry every couple of hours. That only happens when we are metabolically inflexible, incapable of accessing our stored body fat for energy. Based on the research, our natural ancestral pattern is to eat one big meal a day.

Migraines are more likely to begin during sleep than wakefulness, as many migraine sufferers can attest. And more often than not, the migraines that begin during sleep are the worst of the worst. But, we can significantly reduce the likelihood that a migraine will occur during sleep if we ensure that our last meal has been fully digested and metabolized by the time our head hits the pillow.

In other words, we want our body to be back to its physiologic baseline by the time we go to sleep.

One way to achieve this is to adopt an "eating window," a strategy that many folks I've worked with have used to great effect. Here, you choose a particular window of time to eat, usually in the range of 6 to 12 hours. For example, someone who's using a 10-hour window and going to bed at 10 pm might eat their first bite of food at 8 am, and their last one at 6 pm.

The longer you stay on a ketogenic diet, the easier it will be to adhere to a shorter eating window. So, you may want to set a longer eating window at the beginning (10, or even12 hours, for example), and shrink it down over time.

Another option is only to eat while the sun is up so that your window changes with the seasons. Eating only during daylight may be the most evolutionarily appropriate strategy, as research indicates that this was likely how our ancestors did it for hundreds of thousands of years (our three meals a day routine is a very recent cultural "invention"). As a result, eating during daytime is what our bodies still "expect" us to be doing.

6) Eat starchy vegetables (turnips, parsnips, carrots, rutabaga, beets) in moderation, and always as part of a more substantial meal.

Humans have been eating underground root vegetables for a very long time. As such, we can digest them well, and so they can be considered human food. However, given that they are higher in carbohydrates than meat (which is zero carb) and other plant foods (non-starchy vegetables, as above), they shouldn't be a dietary staple for someone trying to achieve nutritional ketosis.

7) **Drink water, coffee, or herbal tea.**

Water should be the primary liquid you drink. In the initial transition into ketosis, adding a pinch of sea salt is a good idea to help replace lost minerals.

Coffee is fine in moderation (1-2 cups per day) with or without heavy cream, but not within 8 hours of bedtime, as a minimum. Drink herbal teas as desired (true teas, which are derived from the tea plant, can be problematic for some, and are best avoided until Phase 3 or 4).

(**RELATED:** If you'd like ideas for what to eat, remember that we have delicious and, most importantly, battle-tested recipes and a first month meal plan available in the free supplemental guide to the book).

CARB COUNTS & MACRONUTRIENT RATIOS

At this point, those of you who are somewhat familiar with the ketogenic diet may be wondering what your daily carb count should be. Or what ratios of fat, protein, and carbs (i.e., macronutrients) you should be eating.

Traditionally, carb counts and macronutrient ratios have been the primary focus of ketogenic diet instructions. It's all about getting the macros right, with little to no attention given to what foods you eat to get there.

Again, that's a mistake. That's why the *Keto for Migraine* guidelines first cover specific foods.

And here's the great thing - just by following the guidelines above, most folks will achieve ketosis, without ever having to busy themselves with carb counts or macronutrient ratios. Essentially, what I've outlined in the guidelines above is the template for the human diet, with some modest adjustments to help make keeping carb intake in the ketogenic range.

That being said, it can be a good idea to monitor daily carbohydrate intake in the beginning. Monitoring is a good idea, especially if you've never paid much attention to the carb counts of the foods you eat, as building this kind of knowledge will be a great asset going forward. You'll probably be surprised by how many carbs can be in "healthy" foods.

There are some of you reading this who will prefer more rigid guidelines and structure, and who actually enjoy counting and tracking carbs (you know who you are). If that's you, feel free to go to town tracking carbs.

HOW MANY CARBS PER DAY?

While it is true that whether or not you stimulate ketosis depends on the amount of dietary carbohydrates you eat, there are also many other factors as well. These include your age, gender, degree of metabolic flexibility, muscle mass, activity level, meal frequency, and even when you eat your carbs and what you eat them with.

For example, whereas a muscular 23-year-old athlete may be able to eat 150 grams of carbs per day and remain in ketosis, a sedentary 65-year-old who's been eating a standard Western diet for decades may require under 20 grams per day. Even then, it may take some time for her keto engine to start firing on all cylinders.

The standard recommendation has been to restrict carbs to between 20 and 50 grams per day, as that's a range that will work for most. But how closely do you need to track your carbs?

Here are a couple of suggested approaches for how to implement the guidelines:

Approach #1: Start with just the seven guidelines listed above, especially if you already have some awareness of the amount of carbs in various foods. If you find that you aren't registering any ketones in the urine after a couple of weeks of eating this way (we'll talk about measuring ketones soon), you can start tracking carbs, and aim to keep them under 50 grams.

Though if you're feeling great and keeping The Beast away, you may not wish to bother - there are many ways in which eating like this helps to protect against The Beast besides the production of ketones, a topic we'll address in a later chapter.

If you still aren't registering ketones after a week or two of restricting carbs to under 50 grams, then reduce them to under 20 grams.

Approach #2: If you've never really looked at the carb counts in food before, then doing some tracking, in the beginning, is a good idea, as this will be useful knowledge going forward. So, in addition to adhering to the primary guidelines above, also aim to keep daily carbs under 50 grams.

If you still aren't registering ketones after a week or two of restricting carbs to under 50 grams, then reduce them to under 20 grams.

MACRONUTRIENT RATIOS
- should you care?

In the early days of keto, it was all about your ratio of fats to carbs to protein. The traditional guidelines were for fat to comprise 70% of our daily calories, protein 25%, and carbs 5%.

The reality is that there's nothing magical about these ratios, which is something that those of us working with lots of keto clients have learned over the past few years. In reality, there's a range of ratios that can work for a single person, and there's a good deal of variability in the ratios that work from one person to the next.

What those of us who've been using ketogenic diets with patients have discovered is that, in most cases, worrying about ratios is again more trouble than it's worth. It's overkill.

That said, if making spreadsheets and tracking details is your idea of a good time, have at it. Just don't get too anxious about it. But, for most, tracking ratios isn't necessary for success.

Now, for a tiny minority of people, tracking ratios may be helpful. So, here's the final rule of thumb: if you still aren't registering ketones after restricting carbs to 20 grams or less for a week or two, then it's worth tracking your macronutrient intake (protein, carbs, and fat) and calculating your ratios. In the vast majority of instances, the problem is going to be not enough fat in the diet (and too much protein). So, the solution will be to increase fat in the diet.

MEASURING KETONES

As we've discussed, one objective of the ketogenic diet is to stimulate the liver to produce ketones. The liver releases them into the blood, and the kidneys ultimately filter them into the urine. By definition, we are in ketosis when there are ketones in the blood.

One convenient thing here is that this is something we can measure with tools that are now readily available. We can look for ketones in our blood or our urine to determine whether or not we've achieved ketosis.

Do you have to measure them? Not necessarily.

Part of whether you should measure just depends on the kind of person you are.

Some people want to know what to do and then not give it a second thought.

Others like to know all the fine details. They want to measure, monitor and quantify.

Some people won't keep a headache diary, no matter how many times I mention it. But occasionally someone brings back 200 pages of spreadsheet data with records of their every waking minute.

You probably know which boat you fall into.

My goal when advocating for any change in diet and lifestyle is to provide the most frictionless path possible so that you can reap the maximum result for the least expenditure of effort. And to make it sustainable. What you do beyond that should be because you want to, not because you feel as if you have to.

For many, by simply adhering to the seven parameters of the *Keto for Migraine* diet, you'll reap the vast majority of the benefits, without any need for testing. As I've said, most people will achieve ketosis by merely following the initial set of guidelines outlined above.

That said, there may be certain circumstances where testing can be of use. These include:

Peace of Mind / Satisfying Curiosity. There is something gratifying about getting official confirmation that the changes you've made are working and that your body is responding as it should. For some, that extra peace of mind is worth it.

Troubleshooting. There may be instances where you need feedback to know if you're on the right track, or if you need to alter what you're doing a bit. Reasons for this would include extended transitional symptoms (fatigue, cramps, mental fogginess lasting beyond the first week) or stalled progress.

Correlating Symptoms with Confirmed Ketosis. Most folks with experience eating a ketogenic diet learn to recognize the body's signals that they've entered ketosis. Those signals can include a surge in energy and mental clarity, a particular taste in the mouth (sweet for some, metallic for others), and other signs.

If you're able to cultivate an awareness of these signs, then you'll be able to use them as a marker going forward, obviating the need for blood or urine testing. Because I've correlated specific physical symptoms with ketone levels, I personally now have a pretty good general idea of whether I'm in ketosis at any given time.

Overall, if you're the type that enjoys self-experimentation, who likes data, and who likes to track and monitor things, then you'll probably enjoy monitoring ketone levels. Also, if you fall into that camp, you'll probably prefer the precision that comes with measuring ketones in the blood (and likewise find the imprecision of urine monitoring unsatisfying).

With that in mind, here are the two primary recommended methods for testing, including how they work, and their advantages and disadvantages. You'll find the links to the strips and blood testing device we like in the Supplemental Guide to *Keto for Migraine* (ketoformigraine.com/guide).

KETONE TESTING METHOD #1: Keto Test Strips (urine)

Advantages:

- Less expensive

- Easy to use

- Easier to find (can get at the drugstore)

- Painless!

Disadvantages:

- Not suitable for tracking precise ketone levels. The urine test is mainly useful for knowing *whether you're in ketosis or not*, but not the degree, or "depth," of ketosis. For this reason, I don't recommend obsessing too much over the color of the strip, only whether or not it looks like you're in the range of ketosis.

- May turn negative after you've been in ketosis for a while (false-negative results).

How to test: Collect urine in a receptacle of some sort and dip the test strip, or hold the strip in your urine stream.

Wait about a minute, check the color, and compare it to the reference colors on the container.

KETONE TESTING METHOD #2: Precision Xtra Monitor (blood)

For ketone monitoring, the gold standard right now is the Precision Xtra device. It can measure either ketones or glucose in the blood and which result you get depends on which test strip you use.

So you'll want to make sure you're getting the ketone strips for testing, which are unfortunately more expensive (i.e., don't get the glucose strips).

Advantages:

- Can get precise ketone levels, and know with certainty whether you're in ketosis

- Will remain positive as long as you're in ketosis

Disadvantages:

- More expensive

- More steps involved

- Not as widely available

- Blood must be spilled!

How to test: Place ketone strip in the monitor (it will automatically turn on and say "ketone" on the display).

Prick fingertip (go towards the edge rather than the middle, where there are fewer nerve endings) with pricking device. Squeeze out an ample drop of blood if need be. Touch the edge of the strip to drop of blood, allowing it to wick upwards until the monitor beeps, indicating the sample is adequate.

The result will display on the screen.

NAVIGATING THE TRANSITION

As we've discussed, there are a whole host of changes that are set in motion when you begin eating this way - changes that have to occur for your body to start producing ketones. Changes that go all the way down to your DNA. Changes that allow you to shift from being a sugar burner to a fat and ketone burner, or to become "keto-adapted."

That change doesn't happen overnight. There's a transitional period as your body moves through those changes, lasting anywhere from a few days to a couple of weeks. Some folks may experience new symptoms during this transitional period. You may hear this referred to as the "keto flu." The intensity of that experience will depend in large part on your diet before eating this way.

If you are moving from a diet that's already low in carbohydrate, the transitional symptoms will likely be minimal. If you are moving from a diet that's higher in carbohydrate, they may be more pronounced.

We've learned a lot in recent years about how to minimize these transitional symptoms, thanks to all the Beast Slaying Keto-Nauts (I just made that word up) who've gone before you.

I consider there to be four major changes that are occurring in the body during this transitional phase. And it is these four changes that explain the five primary transitional symptoms that may arise after initially adopting a ketogenic diet, which are fatigue, hunger, muscle cramps, headaches, and constipation.

Now, it's important to note that many people experience *none* of these. I say that to help ensure you don't fall victim to the nocebo effect (the placebo effect's evil twin, where the expectation of a negative outcome makes that outcome more likely to occur).

But, even if you do experience one of them, you needn't suffer helplessly. In fact, you can usually eliminate (or even prevent) them entirely. Below are the four major changes, how they're connected to the five primary symptoms, and how you can use this knowledge to address any symptom you might experience.

CHANGE #1: THE ENERGY GAP (EG).

Remember that during the transitional phase, the body is moving from sugar/glucose to fat and ketones as its primary fuel source. Multiple changes, which occur on different time scales, must occur for that to happen.

During this time, when dietary carbs (the fuel you've been dependent on) are low, and your fat-burning abilities aren't yet optimized, your brain may sense that there's less energy available to power your body. When the brain senses there's less energy around, you typically feel fatigued and hungry. Fatigue is the brain's way of ensuring that you use less energy, and hunger is the brain's way of ensuring that you consume more energy.

CHANGE #2: FLUID SHIFTS (FS)

The more carbs we eat, the more water we retain. In other words, carbs cause bloating.

When you eat fewer carbs, your body gets rid of that water (you pee it out). You also lose some of the minerals that the water contains (i.e., "electrolytes").

This loss of water and minerals can lead to fatigue, muscle cramps, and headaches.

CHANGE #3: GLYCOGEN DEPLETION (GD)

Our muscles store glucose in a molecule known as glycogen, which we can burn for short bursts of energy. Reducing carbs in the diet can lower our stores of glycogen (especially in the beginning), which can lead to muscle fatigue and cramping. Dehydration can amplify this effect.

Ultimately, as our muscles become well adapted to using fat and ketones, this resolves.

CHANGE #4: DIGESTIVE ADAPTATION

Any time we change our eating habits, our digestive system takes time to adapt. During this adaptation, we may experience a change in our bowel habits. This change can go in either direction - some may experience an increase in stool frequency, and some may experience a reduction (which tends to be the more common response).

I hesitate to use the terms "diarrhea" or "constipation" to describe either of these since we think of those as pathological or problematic conditions when it's more accurate to think of this as a natural and necessary response to a change in our eating habits.

What to do?

Okay, now that we've reviewed the four major changes occurring in the body during the transition to keto, we can know what to do should we experience any of the five primary transitional symptoms (in addition to how to prevent them in the first place).

POSSIBLE SYMPTOM: Fatigue

Potential causes: Energy Gap, Fluid Shifts, and Glycogen Depletion

Remedies:

1) Eat more.

In many cases, eating more will take care of the problem. Remember, during this transition, your body hasn't fully learned how to mobilize and burn your stored body fat.

Until that happens, you're more reliant on food for energy. Increasing the amount of carbs in the diet would be counter-productive. So what to do instead? Increase the amount of fat in the diet.

2) Add MCT or coconut oil.

Medium Chain Triglycerides (MCTs) are a special class of fat, found in highest abundance in coconuts. They're special because they can be a) absorbed very quickly and easily in the liver circulation, and b) converted directly to ketones in the liver once they're there.

Because of those properties, when you eat coconut, coconut oil, or MCT oil, your brain gets a quick hit of ketones, which it can use for energy. Once you've made it through the transition, you'll be generating your own ketones by burning your stored body fat. But, until then, coconut or MCT oil can be used as a bridge.

3) Increase water and mineral intake.

Water is by far the best thing to drink. However, during the transitional period, it can be helpful to add some minerals (aka "salts") to your water to help replace those as well.

There are multiple approaches you can take here. You can add a pinch of sea salt to the water you drink. You can take an electrolyte supplement in pill form. Or you can purchase electrolyte solutions to mix into your water (again, the one I now use after a few years of testing is in the supplemental guide).

POSSIBLE SYMPTOM #2: Hunger

Potential Causes: Energy Gap.

Remedies:

1) **Eat more!** (see details above)

2) **Increase fluid and mineral intake** (see details above), as sometimes dehydration intensifies hunger pangs.

POSSIBLE SYMPTOM #3: Muscle cramping

Potential Causes: Glycogen Depletion, Fluid Shifts

Remedies:

1) **Increase water and mineral intake.** In addition to the recommendations above, taking a Magnesium supplement (400mg) at bedtime can also be helpful, as muscle cramps tend to occur during sleep (see the supplemental guide for the Magnesium supplement we use).

2) **Slow down the rate of carbohydrate reduction.** If cramps remain a significant issue despite increasing water and mineral intake, then consider slowing down the pace of carb reduction. Instead of restricting carbs to the ketogenic range (20-50 grams per day) right away, taper them down over two to three weeks (example: 125 grams in week 1, 100 grams in week 2, 75 grams in week 3).

POSSIBLE SYMPTOM #4: Headaches

Potential Causes: Fluid Shifts

Remedies:

1) Increase water and mineral intake.

The vast majority of headaches that occur during the transitional phase appear to be due to water and mineral losses, as described above. The character of the headache is different than that of a typical migraine - it is usually described as more diffuse (i.e., the whole head), dull, and mild to moderate in intensity.

Since we began recommending that folks add salt to their water during the transitional period, we've virtually stopped hearing about this as an issue.

POSSIBLE SYMPTOM #5: Change in bowel habits

Potential Causes: Digestive Adaptation

Remedies:

Since a reduction in the frequency of bowel movements is the most common issue (again, I hesitate to use the term "constipation," since that implies a pathological condition), that's what I'll focus on in this remedies section.

1) Time. As mentioned, a change in bowel habits is a necessary and expected adaptation to a change in eating habits. Given the tight link between eating and digestion, it would be quite surprising if this didn't change after we made a significant change to our diet.

2) MCT oil. As already mentioned, MCT oil can be helpful during the transition to ketosis by supplying a quick burst of ketones (when I've used it, I usually add maybe a teaspoon to my morning coffee). MCT oil can also be used for constipation, as it can help speed up transit through the lower GI tract. A little can go a long way here, so it's best to start with a small amount and increase gradually to your desired effect (to avoid any bathroom "emergencies.").

Additionally, avoid taking MCT oil if you have a migraine (more on the reasons why later).

3) Flaxseed. A little bit of flaxseed (usually sprinkled on top of something) can also help speed things along.

As mentioned, these are all symptoms that occur during the transition to nutritional ketosis. By definition, they are transient.

Once the transition is complete and you've ramped up your fat-burning capabilities and adapted to using ketones as fuel, you'll more than likely experience the polar opposite of these symptoms.

Fatigue will be replaced by a surge in energy levels (for many, this will be energy unlike anything they've experienced since they were kids). Gone will be the post-lunchtime sleep attack that's the bane of the nine-to-fiver's existence.

The ravenous hunger typically experienced between meals will evaporate, and you'll likely be astounded at your ability to go extended periods without feeling like you have to eat.

And, of course, you probably wouldn't be reading this if you hadn't already heard you might experience a radical reduction in visitations from The Beast!

HOW LONG?

So just how long should you do this keto thing? There are two questions to answer here.

First, how long should you do keto to conduct an adequate keto experiment? And the second, if your keto experiment is going really, really well, how long should you stay on keto? Or how about just staying keto forever?

Let's tackle the first question.

One of our objectives with our keto experiment is to collect data. To understand how you respond to a keto diet. To understand what it *feels like* to be in ketosis.

As we've already discussed, your body experiences a significant transition when first moving into ketosis. This switch unfolds over time, with various stages that occur over multiple durations. A lot of that change happens early on, within the first couple days to a couple of weeks.

That said, research on those who've been keto for years has demonstrated that changes still occur years into a ketogenic diet, primarily concerning the efficiency with which the body burns fat.

By and large, however, we can view the transition as mostly completed after the first two weeks. As such, we know we need more time than that to conduct an adequate self-experiment. And it also means that those first two weeks are not the time to be collecting data about the impact of ketosis on ourselves. During that time, we're learning about how we experience the *transition* into ketosis.

My typical recommendation over the years has been to set a minimum of 30 days. That translates to about two weeks of stable ketosis for most folks. Still not a lot of time, but enough for most people to experience some indication of how they feel while they're in ketosis.

For migraineurs, that of course includes how their head feels.

And here are three possible outcomes that you may experience, along with guidelines for considering how to proceed.

Outcome 1: You're doing better.

You're feeling great all the way around, and you've detected a positive impact on your migraines. In our experience over the past few years, this is by far the most common result. Not surprisingly, those who experience this outcome generally have no desire to stop doing keto. In this case, your question will almost inevitably be, "how long can I continue to do this?" or "is there a reason I should ever stop?"

I'll address that question in just a minute.

Outcome 2: You haven't noticed a change one way or another.

You may have seen some positive changes like [desired] weight loss, improved energy, or mental clarity, but you haven't noticed a discernible change in your migraines.

Here, it makes sense to continue. Based on all of the evidence we have, it is likely that keto has moved you closer to where you want to be.

And, improvements with migraine rarely happen linearly but are rather stepwise. Meaning there are periods of stability punctuated by bursts of improvement, where your efforts build up to a critical threshold that finally pays dividends.

In other words, in many cases with migraines, progress is occurring beneath the surface before it becomes evident to us. Remember the story of bamboo.

Furthermore, as mentioned earlier, the metabolic adaptations to keto continue for quite some time after initiating a ketogenic diet. The longer we maintain it, the larger the potential benefit. If we stop, we lose out on this accumulation of benefit.

Outcome 3: You're feeling worse.

This is the least likely scenario. As I've discussed, arguably the most common reason this happens is that someone adopts a migraine-unfriendly version of keto. So, that shouldn't happen to you.

The other common reason is that the impact of abortive medications is still playing a major role.

Remember that the abortive medications are a "zero multiplier." In other words, their effects can neutralize all of other efforts to thwart The Beast, including keto.

This is why I recommend folks wait till they're in Phase 2 or higher on the Timeline of Migraine Freedom before adopting keto, primarily to ensure that the abortive meds won't undermine their success (or present the illusion that keto doesn't help).

In this scenario, I think it makes the most sense to stop keto after the 30-day trial and instead focus on implementing the other aspects of The Migraine Miracle plan that build the 3 Pillars of Protection (and building these up does not require you to be keto).

In many cases, re-trying the keto experiment after doing so results in a much better outcome. How? Because those changes you've made have now put you in a place where you can reap the benefits of keto.

Remember, we are continually changing creatures. We're not the same person today we were yesterday, all the way down to the genes that are active or inactive. So, how we respond to something six months from now may be quite different than how we respond today.

Keto has been such a life-changing tool for so many that **I'd hate to see anyone wrongly conclude that it wasn't for them simply because the timing (or execution) wasn't right.**

Okay, now for the second question - for those who are feeling fantastic, how long can you stay on keto?

Or, put another way, should you ever stop?

It makes perfect sense. You're feeling better than you've felt in years, maybe several decades, so it may seem crazy to think of ever doing things differently. Why mess with a good thing?

If you find yourself in this situation, you mainly want to know if are there any drawbacks to being in ketosis long term.

The truth is that nobody can answer that question definitively. We don't know for sure because it would require longitudinal studies on people who've been keto over long periods. The best data of that nature that we have comes from patients treated for epilepsy with a ketogenic diet - here we have patients who've been on it for over five years who show no adverse effects.

That's not to say we can't make reasonable and scientifically-backed predictions about long term ketosis.

Along those lines, what might we be concerned about regarding eating a ketogenic diet long term?

One thing might be your nutritional needs - can a ketogenic diet provide all the nutrients we need over the long term? After all, we were told for decades that the foundation of a healthy diet were grains and carbohydrates. Which is odd because carbohydrate-rich foods tend to be the least nutrient-dense foods we have. To get the same amount of nutrients from carbohydrate-rich foods requires we eat more calories - one reason why diets high in carbs are so fattening.

What are the most nutrient-dense foods we have? Animal foods and non-starchy plants. Both of these are nutritional power-houses.

Animal foods have the added advantage in that we can digest and absorb those nutrients much better since plant foods contain substances that block nutrient absorption. For example, while beef and grains both contain iron, we absorb around 400% more of the iron in beef than the iron in grains (those 20 grams of iron in a cup of rice bran does us zero good if it doesn't make it into our body).

In other words, when we remove high-carb foods from our diet and replace them with lower-carb ones, we are significantly *increasing* the amount of nutrients in our diet. This disparity is amplified even further if we add in organ meats, the most nutrient-dense foods of all.

Thus, nutrient deficiencies are less likely to occur on a ketogenic diet that follows the guidelines outlined in this chapter (this is in contrast to plant-based diets, where nutritional supplementation is a must to prevent serious vitamin deficiencies and brain dysfunction). As mentioned, the nutritional value of the diet can be increased even further through the regular consumption of organ meats (liver, kidney, heart) in addition to a variety of non-starchy plants, both of which are encouraged.

Another thing you may wonder about with long-term keto is whether there are drawbacks to remaining in that metabolic state for long periods. Certainly, we have no reason to fear ketones themselves. On the contrary, we continue to learn about their health-giving benefits.

Some have argued that a long term ketogenic diet may also lead to metabolic inflexibility. If you recall, being metabolically flexible means you can readily shift between burning sugar/glucose or fat for fuel. On the standard high-carb Western diet, most people are dependent on carbohydrates for energy because they cannot mobilize and burn stored body fat when it's needed.

But, metabolic inflexibility can work in the opposite direction. Prolonged carbohydrate restriction can conceivably lead to the body reducing its sugar burning machinery so that you become a less effective sugar burner. In this scenario, you can't switch from burning fats to burning sugar as readily.

Yet, this is a reversible situation, and reflects a smart adaptation on the part of your body (again, why keep sugar burning machinery around when you're not using it). The primary scenario where this would be problematic is for high-level athletes involved in sports where this kind of metabolic flexibility is advantageous. So, while this variant of metabolic inflexibility may compromise athletic performance in a very small minority, there is no evidence to support or reason to believe that it compromises *health*.

Returning to our original question - are there any drawbacks to long term ketosis? None that we know of, and no compelling reason to believe there would be. In fact, given what we know today, it's harder to make the argument for why we *shouldn't* be in ketosis long term. Because, by all accounts, running our body on glucose is more damaging than running it on ketones.

My personal concerns about long-term ketosis are close to zero. If you want to play it safe, you can simply cycle in and out of ketosis periodically. Two months on, one month off. Three weeks on, one week off. There are many options here, and no right or wrong way.

Or, you can do as I do, and let the rhythms of nature be your guide for when to eat plant foods (fresh fruits and vegetables). If you do so, then you'll naturally go very low carb in the winter months, which is probably the most evolutionarily appropriate way of all to do it.

It's important to remember that **ketosis is a natural physiological state.** It's something our body is designed to do.

Given what we know of their lifestyles and habitats, our wild human ancestors likely spent a large chunk of their lives in ketosis. In nature, human foods that are higher in carbohydrates are most abundant in the summer months and virtually non-existent in the colder months. If humans didn't continue to thrive while in ketosis, we'd have long ago gone extinct, and you wouldn't be reading this book right now!

From this perspective, asking if keto is harmful over the long term is akin to asking if breathing air is dangerous over the long term.

Lastly, there may be some of you who wish to stop keto for a while but worry about the consequences. You've experienced an amazing transformation, and don't want to mess things up. Maybe there are certain foods you miss, ones you'd like to add back into your diet.

If you find yourself in this situation, you mainly want to know if going out of keto will cause you to regress to where you were before you started.

The good news: that's very unlikely, and there are multiple reasons why. First, as we've discussed, **you are not the same person after keto that you were before keto.** You've transcribed new genes, built a new set of metabolic machinery, likely shed some excess body fat and added more lean tissue, and so on.

Second, it's not like you'll be going back to eating the standard Western diet, gorging on sugar, grains, and packaged convenience foods. Now that you've experienced first hand the intimate connection between food and health, that seems like a ridiculous idea.

Instead, you'll still be sticking to the basic principles of the

Migraine Miracle plan. And more than likely, you'll be much further down the Timeline of Migraine Freedom now that you've built up your 3 Pillars of Protection.

We've worked with many people in this situation, and I don't know of a single one who regressed to where they started from after going out of keto.

Remember, a ketogenic diet isn't necessary for building the 3 Pillars of Protection against migraine. For migraines, I view keto as a tool for accelerating progress to migraine freedom (while providing a host of other benefits). So, while it can help you get where you want to go faster, it usually isn't necessary to keep you there.

One final caveat - if and when you do decide to stop keto, a slow exit is advisable. In other words, don't go from 30 to 100 daily carbs in a single day. Instead, try gradually increasing your daily carbs (by around 10-20 grams per day) until you reach your desired baseline diet. Most everyone will end up finding their carbohydrate threshold beyond which they feel worse (lower energy, mental fogginess, headaches, etc.), which in our experience tends to be somewhere between 80 and 130 carbs per day (higher for those who are very active).

KEYS FROM CHAPTER 4:

1) Attending to all 3 Pillars of Protection against The Beast is the key to success with a ketogenic diet for the migraineur.

2) When migraineurs don't see progress with keto, it's usually due to either the continued impact of abortive medications or the consumption of non-

human-but-technically-still-keto foods.

3) For most, just adhering to the seven guidelines to *Keto for Migraine* is sufficient to reap the benefits.

4) In some instances, tracking daily carb intake is beneficial. In rare cases, tracking and adhering to specific macronutrient (fats, carbs, and protein) ratios is helpful.

CHAPTER 5: MAXIMIZING FOR WEIGHT GAIN (& LOSS)

WHAT YOU'LL LEARN IN THIS CHAPTER: The keto-genic diet is arguably the single best way to lose fat - and to do so without suffering. So good that the most common question I get from those on the Keto for Migraine plan is how to gain weight.

In this chapter, we'll begin by clarifying the confusion around the topic of weight and body fat. And then you'll learn strategies for both maximizing weight gain or weight loss on the Keto for Migraine plan.

It's almost a certainty that you're aware that the ketogenic diet is great for anyone who wants to lose weight.

And it's easy to understand why it works so well. As we've learned, in order to reach nutritional ketosis, we must be burning a certain amount of body fat.

Number one, the diet stimulates the release of fat from our fat tissues. Releasing this fat is the only way we can sustain nutritional ketosis. **Exactly what we want when we're trying to lose weight.** The longer we stay on it, the better we become at mobilizing and burning our stored body fat.

Being able to access stored body fat for energy when we need it means we no longer have to eat every couple of hours to avoid getting hangry. Even better, ketones themselves suppress appetite.

This is why the ketogenic has gone viral. It *works*.

Does every single person lose weight on a ketogenic diet? No.

But when desired weight loss doesn't happen, it's almost always because of the kinds of foods being eaten. Just as with *Keto for Migraine*, diet quality does matter for weight loss, too (just not quite as much, and with less painful consequences).

It's exceedingly rare for someone who's adhering to the *Keto for Migraine* guidelines outlined in chapter 4 to not shed excess body fat or lose weight. So much so that **the question that we've gotten way more often over the years is not how to lose weight on keto, but how to *gain* it.**

So, if you find yourself losing more weight on keto than you'd like, here are some recommendations on what to do (and for those of you who want to maximize the weight loss benefits of keto, I'll get to that next).

HOW TO GAIN WEIGHT ON A KETOGENIC DIET (if you dare...)

As I said, the ketogenic diet is excellent for shedding excess body fat. But what if you notice your weight dropping more than you'd like? What if you find yourself dropping weight you didn't want to lose?

Bodyweight is a murky and complicated topic. There's much confusion, misconception, and mythology surrounding it, so let's begin by clearly defining what it is we're talking about.

First, we need to clarify what we mean when we refer to body weight. One of the problems here is that "weight" is an imprecise term, and measuring and monitoring bodyweight alone can lead to misleading information.

Our total body weight is the sum total of all the "stuff" that we're made of. We can break that "stuff" into categories, which are:

- Organ weight
- "Lean" tissue (muscles, tendons, bones) weight
- Body fat
- Water (most of our weight is water)

Expressed mathematically, **Total Body Weight = Organ Weight + Lean Tissue Weight + Body Fat + Water**

When the numbers change on the scale, we're only getting the net sum of those four categories. Though we can make an educated guess at it, we can't know where that change came from just by looking at the scale.

Again, when we gain or lose weight, that gain or loss can come from any of that stuff. And when we talk about wanting to "gain" or "lose" weight, we really must specify what stuff we actually want to gain or lose, because how we go about it will differ according to the stuff we're trying to add or lose.

When we say we want to "lose weight," for example, what we really mean is that we want to lose body fat. We're not interested in losing parts of our bones or organs.

And when we say we want to "gain weight," what we actually

mean is that we want to gain muscle (in rare situations, we may want to gain body fat as well).

We can change the amount of body fat, water, and lean tissue we have. Our body protects organ mass, so our organ tissue will only be broken down as a last resort (in cases of extreme malnutrition). So if we want to lose or gain weight, we can gain that weight in the form of fat, muscle, or water.

And regardless of whether we want to gain or lose, it's essential first to ask why do we want to do so, and second, what "stuff" do we want to gain or lose. Do we want to gain or lose fat, water, or lean tissue (muscles, bones, and other structural components)?

Often when people mention wanting to gain weight, there's not a compelling reason why other than a nebulous worry about being too thin, or pressure from obtrusive friends and family.

The primary health reasons for wanting to gain weight would be a loss of lean body mass due to insufficient protein intake (i.e., the body is forced to break down its own parts to meet protein requirements), or extremely low body fat to a degree that it impacts the endocrine system (which is very rare).

I wouldn't personally embark down the road of trying to add more weight (in the name of better health, at least) unless I had clear evidence that one of these two things was happening.

I understand there may be other motivations (cosmetic, cultural norms, etc.), but it's crucial to recognize that those motivations aren't moving us towards better health. In other words, our appearance, or simply being outside of the bell curve of the "normal" population, wouldn't be a *health* reason for wanting to gain weight.

So back to the original question - *if* you are eating keto and are thinking you want to gain weight, *and* you've assessed your reasons for wanting to do so and find them compelling, then here's how I would go about it.

First, decide on what kind of stuff you want to add to your body. While there are four categories of "stuff" that contribute to weight, only two of those are modifiable when eating low carb (since we can't do much to modify organ mass, and since retaining more water would require that we increase our carbohydrate intake).

So we have two possible places where we can add "weight."

1. Lean tissue.
2. Body fat.

If you want to add more lean tissue, the primary means by which you can do is to add more muscle. To add muscle, we must do two things. First, we must stimulate the muscles to grow. And second, we must provide our muscles with the raw materials they need for growth.

We stimulate muscle growth through physical activity, and resistance/weight training in particular (moving the muscles against resistance). **Resistance exercise creates the *demand* for growth.**

After that, we must give our muscles the raw materials for growth through dietary protein. As you may know, too much protein can potentially knock you out of ketosis; however, physical activity and resistance exercise will tend to raise the threshold where that occurs (i.e., the greater the demands on your muscles, and the greater your muscle mass, the more protein you can eat and remain in ketosis).

If you want to add more body fat, on the other than hand, then you must eat more food. Now, one of the typical advantages of a ketogenic diet is improved appetite regulation. Unlike on the standard Western high-carb diet, our brain isn't telling us to eat more than we need to meet our current energy needs.

This restoration of our satiety system means that most people tend to spontaneously eat fewer calories on a ketogenic diet, likely for several reasons. So you'll have to figure out a way to get in more food so that those excess calories will be stored away as fat.

My recommendation for doing so is to find something that's still within the *Keto for Migraine* set of guidelines that you find especially delicious. Something that you might continue eating even after you're full.

In technical terms, foods that we continue to eat even when no longer hungry are labeled as "hyper-palatable." Most every packaged convenience food that comes in a box or bag has been precisely designed to be hyper-palatable. So, identify what *Keto for Migraine* compliant foods (or recipes) meet that criterion for you (or try to find them), and eat more of them.

Again, I think there are very few situations that merit deliberate attempts to gain weight (though engaging in regular resistance exercise to build strength is undoubtedly a worthwhile endeavor). So, before proceeding along these lines, make sure you've thought about it very carefully, are very clear on *why* you're doing it, are clear on the type of "weight" you're trying to add, and are confident that the benefits outweigh the **downsides**.

HOW TO MAXIMIZE WEIGHT LOSS ON A KETOGENIC DIET: KFM + TRE = MAXIMAL FAT LOSS

Okay, what about weight loss?

Maybe you have some extra pounds you'd like to shed, and you want to maximize your efforts to do so. Or perhaps you've been keto for a bit and aren't noticing any drop in body fat.

Or maybe you've been keto and have noticed the scale going in the wrong direction.

As mentioned, most who adopt the *Keto for Migraine* (KFM) plan don't typically have issues losing weight. That's why we get far more questions about how to gain weight than how to lose it.

And that's because the plan sticks to eating real, evolutionarily appropriate food. It's the ketogenic diet for humans.

Where most folks run into trouble, as we've discussed, is in eating a ketogenic diet that's not appropriate for humans. Above, I mentioned that eating "hyper-palatable" foods was the key strategy for adding body fat - these are foods that you find hard to stop eating even when you're no longer hungry.

As you might imagine, if someone's version of a keto diet consists primarily of hyper-palatable foods (and many of the keto recipes on the internet and keto diet books include lots of these), then losing body fat will be a challenge. And in some cases, this version of keto will lead to weight gain.

This is why the typical internet version of keto is far more likely to lead to less weight loss, or even weight gain, when compared to the *Keto for Migraine* plan.

But, if for whatever reason you find fat loss stalling, or you want to do what you can to accelerate it, here's a nearly foolproof protocol for doing so. It's best to wait till you've made it through the keto transitional phase to adopt this protocol since it involves combining a ketogenic diet with time-restricted eating (i.e., an "eating window").

Step 1: Choose an eating window. Weigh yourself to establish a baseline.

An eating window is just the hours within which you're going to eat each day. A reasonable window to start with is 10 hours. So, for example, if you typically eat your first bite of food at 8 am, then your last bite of food would be no later than 6 pm.

If you've been doing keto or low carb for any length of time (i.e., you've already developed a degree of metabolic flexibility), or have already done some intermittent fasting, you may wish to start with a shorter window, like 8 hours (so an 8-hour window might be 8 am to 4 pm, or 10 am to 6 pm).

Step 2: Every few days, measure ketones before your first meal.

Here, the goal is to measure ketones at the end of your fasting interval. All you're looking to do here is confirm that you're in ketosis.

You can use the urine strips to do so; however, be aware that you may get false negative readings (saying you're not in ketosis when you are) if you've been keto for awhile. So, if you get a positive result, then you're good to go. If you get a negative reading, you might want to try a different monitoring device like the Precision Xtra blood test.

Step 3: After two weeks, weigh yourself.

If you haven't lost anything, or if you're not showing ketones when you check, then reduce your eating window by one to two hours (if you've found your current eating window somewhat challenging, go for one; if not, go for two).

If you've lost weight, keep your same eating window for the next two weeks.

Step 4: Repeat steps 1-3.

Note: If you don't have access to a keto monitor, or don't wish to measure ketones, then you can eliminate step two.

WHY THIS WORKS SO WELL

Why does this work so well for shedding body fat? Because we're essentially combining the two most powerful methods for doing so - nutritional ketosis and time-restricted eating. And **we're combining them in a way that allows us to maximize the impact of both.**

Remember that in order to make ketones, we have to be burning fat for energy above a certain threshold. And we have two sources of fat we can burn - the fat we eat, and the fat we mobilize from our body's stores.

During our fasting window (the time from our last to our first bite of food), we are no longer providing our body with any fat from the diet. This is especially true towards the latter part of our fasting window when that fat from our last meal has long since been digested and metabolized.

So, **if we're in ketosis at the end of our fasting window, we not only know that we're burning lots of fat, we also know that all of that fat has come from our own body.** The only way to be in ketosis at the end of our fasting window is if we're supplying all of the necessary fat from our own stores.

What we're doing here is finding the eating window where this is true, and continuing to adhere to that window until it is no longer true.

Furthermore, intermittent fasting accelerates the establishment of metabolic flexibility. So, this protocol also will continue to stimulate the adaptations that help you readily burn body fat and use ketones for energy.

KEYS TO CHAPTER 5:

1) Bodyweight consists of four different constituents - our organs, body fat, lean tissue, and water.

2) On the *Keto for Migraine* plan, we can modify the weight of our body fat and lean tissue.

3) The best way to gain lean tissue on the *Keto for Migraine* plan is to combine resistance exercise with more dietary protein. The best way to gain body fat is to eat foods you find "hyper-palatable" that are within the *Keto for Migraine* guidelines.

4) Using the *Keto for Migraine* plan with Time Restricted Eating (KFM + TRE) combines our two most powerful tools for weight loss.

CHAPTER 6: HOW KETO HELPS THE MIGRAINE BRAIN

WHAT YOU'LL LEARN IN THIS CHAPTER: It's natural to assume that the benefits of the ketogenic diet are a result of the ketones themselves. Yet, there's likely much more to the story.

In this chapter, you'll learn how the ketones themselves help the migraine brain, along with all the many benefits of the ketogenic diet that have nothing at all to do with ketones!

So how exactly does the ketogenic diet protect us from migraines? While the natural temptation is to attribute all the benefits to the ketones themselves, as you'll see, that's not only a logical error, but a mistake that can sabotage your success with keto.

So, as you folks well know, nutritional ketosis is emerging as a therapeutic tool for a host of neurological conditions, including migraines.

But why?

Why do we believe that the ketogenic diet would be helpful for such things?

Now, this may sound like an academic question — something worthwhile for scientists to figure out, but not something with much practical value.

I think otherwise, and hopefully after this chapter, you'll understand why.

IT'S THE KETONES, RIGHT?

When faced with the question of why nutritional ketosis works so well, what's the natural place to look to try to understand why? At the ketones themselves, of course.

After all, ketosis is defined by the presence of ketones - the molecules acetoacetate and beta-hydroxybutyrate - in the blood. And the whole point of the ketogenic diet is to stimulate our body to make them.

So, understanding why keto works should just be a matter of understanding how ketones affect the body and brain, right? Hold on a second, tiger!

As discussed in earlier chapters, we're making all sorts of changes to our diet and lifestyle when we adopt a ketogenic diet. And those changes impact our body in innumerable ways.

One way it impacts us is that it stimulates our liver to make ketones. The key word in that last sentence being "one way." Because there are all sorts of other things happening, too!

We've already talked about how those changes can spell the difference between a ketogenic diet that propels you down the path to migraine freedom and one that invites The Beast in for a tea party.

What's more, it remains entirely possible that many, even most, of the benefits of nutritional ketosis are a byproduct of those other changes, and not directly related to the ketones themselves.

I'm not suggesting at all that the ketones aren't *part* of the story. There's good evidence to believe that the ketones themselves have some pretty magical effects on our brain, that they do have a role to play.

But here let's consider some of the reasons, ketones and beyond, why a ketogenic diet is such a powerful weapon against The Beast. I think you'll find knowing that it's not all about the ketones, and knowing these other benefits of the ketogenic diet, to be valuable information in many ways.

THE 9 POSSIBLE REASONS KETO FIGHTS MIGRAINES

REASON #1: The elimination (or reduction) of sugar.

It seems that we humans are heavily biased towards attributing an effect to something we've added, or started doing, rather than to something we've taken away, or stopped doing. That's one reason our minds automatically assume that it's the ketones that are providing all the benefits from a ketogenic diet.

But of course it's virtually impossible to stimulate ketone production with any added sugar in the diet. And we surely know that **eliminating sugar is one of the single best things any of us can do to improve our health and to protect against migraines.**

REASON #2: The increase in metabolic flexibility.

We've already discussed that metabolic flexibility is one of the 3 Pillars of Protection against migraine.

And one of the central problems with the standard Western diet is that it makes us metabolically inflexible. It renders us unable to readily shift from burning sugar (i.e., glucose) for energy to burning fat (in this case referring to stored fat from the fat tissues).

Reducing dietary carbs, along with physical activity, are the keys to establishing metabolic flexibility, and a ketogenic diet is a fantastic way to accelerate that process. As discussed, this is precisely why it's becoming the definitive tool for weight loss.

Another reason why switching from carb-centric (burning mainly glucose for energy) to fat-centric metabolism (burning mainly fat for energy) is that **it gets us off of the blood sugar roller coaster,** which is a direct result of a diet high in carbohydrate. These frequent, Beast-provoking daily swings in blood sugar are eliminated on a ketogenic diet.

Many migraineurs report "hunger headaches," or headaches that are brought about when their blood sugar crashes. In my experience, these disappear entirely on a ketogenic diet, even when folks go extended periods of time (16 to 72 hours) without eating. **It's not hunger that's the enemy, it's the erratic metabolic state caused by a diet with far too many carbohydrates.**

REASON #3: Eating less calorically dense foods.

Studies show that those on a keto diet usually eat fewer calories than people on a standard diet. They don't deliberately eat less; it just takes less energy to feel satisfied.

Furthermore, there is evidence that migraines are at least in part triggered and sustained during situations where there's an energy surplus, or when the body has been thrown out of energy equilibrium.

The worst possible kind of foods for throwing us out of energy equilibrium are those that are high in refined carbohydrates since they are energy-dense (lots of calories in a small amount of food) but almost devoid of nutrients.

When moving to a ketogenic diet, not only are you eliminating the worst offenders when it comes to energy-dense foods, you're also reducing the total amount of energy consumed. As a result, the amount of time you're spending in a state of energy surplus, out of energy equilibrium, is reduced.

REASON #4: Better quality sleep.

Many people on a ketogenic diet report improvements in sleep. Specifically, they report a significant reduction in grogginess in the morning (grogginess being a reliable sign of poor sleep), and they report substantial improvements in daytime alertness and energy.

The research, which has shown improvements in sleep quantity and quality on a ketogenic diet, supports these anecdotal reports.

Interestingly, folks in ketosis often note that they need *less* sleep to feel refreshed. Given that one of the primary roles of sleep is to remove the waste generated the prior day from the brain, the fact that burning ketones generates less waste may explain why less sleep could be needed during ketosis.

Virtually every migraineur appreciates the powerful connection between sleep and migraines, and the research here is also quite clear: **anything that improves sleep will fortify the brain against migraines.**

Whether this improvement in sleep is a direct effect of the ketones themselves remains an open question. Regardless, this is another channel by which ketosis protects against the Beast.

REASON #5: Improved mood and reduced anxiety.

Another very promising application of the ketogenic diet is within the realm of mental health. Like most things related to keto, the research on the clinical applications in psychiatry is still in its infancy, but the early studies are favorable.

Yet, psychiatrists and other mental health providers with a holistic approach are already using keto as a primary clinical tool because of the dramatic results they've seen with patients. As has been the case with migraine, responses to a ketogenic diet can far surpass what's possible with the latest pharmaceuticals.

What about the ketogenic diet is causing these improvements? We don't know.

It could be from the anxiety-reducing effects of the ketones themselves. It could be from the stabilization of mood resulting from the removal of refined carbohydrates in the diet. It could be from removing the impact of plant lectins. Plant lectins can disrupt the gut and brain barrier, which can lead to inflammation in the brain. It could be from improvements in brain function due to eating more essential fats (more on that below).

REASON #6: Improvements in gut health.

There is considerable evidence to support a solid connection between the health of the gut and migraines. Conditions that are known to be associated with inflammation and increased permeability of the gut ("leaky gut") are consistently associated with a heightened risk of migraines, a topic I've written and discussed extensively elsewhere (including the "Gluten & Migraine Connection" episode of the Migraine Miracle Moment podcast).

A ketogenic diet requires the elimination of many of the foods known to promote inflammation and leaky gut - sugar and refined carbohydrates, processed foods, and gluten grains.

Removing the biggest gut-disrupting villains means improved defenses against foreign substances entering the bloodstream and reduced systemic (and likely brain) inflammation - both of which are enormously important to the migraineur.

REASON #7: Increased consumption of essential fatty acids.

The brain is mostly fat. Some of those fats our body can make. Some we must obtain from our diet. Research indicates that the most critical of these are the omega-3 fats EPA (eicosapentaenoic acid) and DHA (docosahexaenoic acid).

It's likely that most people eating the high-carb western diet aren't getting enough of these critical compounds. Given how essential they are for brain health, it's brain function that pays the price when our diet is deficient.

Most people who adopt a ketogenic diet will naturally consume more of these essential fats (again, we must replace all those useless calories from refined carbs with something, and that something is going to be fat and protein). Those who make a point to consume more foods rich in EPA and DHA (like eggs and seafood) benefit even more.

REASON #8: The ketones themselves.

It is still well within the realm of possibility that the migraine protective benefits of the ketogenic diet are unrelated to the ketones themselves. That being said, I don't consider that to be very likely. Why?

Because we have evidence that suggests they do confer specific benefits, and because we have multiple biologically plausible ways in which they could exert such an effect.

In an earlier chapter, we discussed how a ketogenic diet results in less oxidative stress in the body and brain, which fits nicely with the emerging theory of migraine as a homeostatic response to oxidative stress.

But, in addition to being a cleaner form of fuel for the brain and protecting against oxidative stress, there are other possible ways in which ketones protect against migraines, including:

1) Increase in inhibitory and decrease in excitatory neurotransmitters. Migraines, seizures, and certain mood disorders have all been associated with an increase in neuronal "excitability." Brain cells communicate with each other by sending electrical signals.

You can think of a "hyper-excitable" brain as one where those signals are sent too readily. Ketones appear to increase the amount of chemicals in the brain (neurotransmitters) that suppress the firing of brain cells ("inhibitory neurotransmitters") and reduce the amount of chemicals in the brain that promote brain cell firing. The net result of this effect on neurotransmitters is to make the brain less "excitable."

2) Reduced inflammation. Inflammation in the brain is a fundamental feature of many neurological disorders. The "white spots" often seen on the MRIs of those with migraine may be a marker of inflammation in the brain caused by the immune system's response to foreign substances.

Ketones have been shown to reduce the inflammatory response of immune cells, which can reduce the amount of inflammation in the brain.

REASON #9: Any number of things we don't know about yet!

At this moment, there is far more that we don't understand about the brain and body than we do understand. And that is certainly true when it comes to the impact of ketones on the brain.

The point is that there's a whole lot of change happening when we go keto, all the way down to the transcription of our DNA. It may be a great many years before we fully understand the nature of those changes and why they make the brain less prone to migraines.

Now, I promised at the beginning of this chapter to explain why understanding this was more than an academic exercise. So why bother pointing out that there are multiple benefits to the ketogenic diet besides the production of ketones?

Because too many times I've seen a person's excessive focus on ketones undermine the benefits of the diet. And this can work in both directions. It's one of several reasons why I don't think measuring for ketones is an absolute necessity. It can be helpful to do so, but only if you're able to maintain perspective.

For example, **just because you aren't showing ketones on your testing device doesn't mean you aren't doing great things for your body and brain.**

Likewise, **just because you are measuring ketones doesn't**

automatically guarantee that good things will happen!

Additionally, I hope that this discussion also illustrates why it would be a mistake to view a ketone *supplement* (like exogenous ketones or MCT oil) as a *replacement* for nutritional ketosis.

Though these may have benefits in special circumstances (like for high-level endurance athletes), it's highly unlikely that these would confer any of the same benefits as nutritional ketosis. And, given that ketone supplements are outside the bounds of our evolutionary experience, they may introduce risks that we've yet to discover.

Hopefully by now I've hammered the point home enough that the ketones themselves are just one of many variables in the overall ketogenic diet equation. And just focusing on the ketones causes us to lose sight of all those other potential benefits. Like the proverb of the blind man and the elephant, if we just focus on a tiny part, we'll never see the big picture!

KEYS FROM CHAPTER 6:

1) While there is evidence that the ketones themselves are part of the reason why a ketogenic diet helps the migraine brain, there are likely many other reasons beyond the ketones.

2) Focusing exclusively on the presence or absence of ketones causes us to lose sight of the many other benefits of the *Keto for Migraine* plan beyond the production of ketones.

3) In other words, don't stress about the ketones!

CHAPTER 7: OTHER BENEFITS OF KETO

WHAT YOU'LL LEARN IN THIS CHAPTER: These are exciting times for the ketogenic diet. Beyond what we already know of its benefits to the brain, the emerging research is indicating that it may transform how we treat all chronic health conditions. In this chapter, we'll briefly cover some of the most exciting areas where the ketogenic diet is showing promise, from brain disorders and beyond.

It's hard not to be enthusiastic about what the future holds for the ketogenic diet. It's already shown itself to be massively more helpful in certain conditions than the most state-of-the-art pharmaceuticals, with none of the significant and unpredictable drawbacks of drugs.

And this is only just the beginning. The floodgates to research on the ketogenic diet have opened, and it seems every day we're learning about some new potential application.

So, I would be remiss if I didn't at least mention some of the other areas where the ketogenic diet is showing great promise as a therapeutic tool. Number one, because knowing this may impact how you choose to use it going forward.

Number two, because it may offer you a means by which to share keto with others you think could benefit from it. If you're like most folks, after experiencing your transformation you're going to want to share it with others you care about so that they too can experience the same.

Given what we already know, I think cycling in and out of ketosis should now be considered as part of the foundation of a healthy lifestyle. Especially for those concerned with protecting the health and function of their brains - which of course should be everyone! But it's becoming increasingly clear that keto has both preventative *and* therapeutic powers.

With that in mind, here's a short overview of some of the areas in health (beyond migraines and epilepsy) where the ketogenic diet is showing great promise as a therapeutic tool.

Cancer. It's long been known that many cancer cells require glucose to survive. Depriving those cells of dietary glucose with a ketogenic diet is a way of selectively killing off the cancerous cells (unlike chemotherapy, which kills cells indiscriminately). Though not limited to this area, the ketogenic diet has shown particular promise in treating brain cancer.

Diabetes. Type 2 diabetes has reached epidemic proportions and is a disease that is a direct consequence of our modern high-carbohydrate diet. The signature problem of type 2 diabetes is that the cells develop resistance to the effects of insulin, resulting in toxic levels of glucose in the blood and widespread organ damage.

A ketogenic diet not only provides an alternative, non-toxic fuel source but has even been shown to reverse the disease altogether. In a study of the ketogenic diet for diabetes treatment performed by Virta Health, 68% of study subjects were able to stop all diabetes medications after one year, and 55% of those who remained on a ketogenic diet for two years reversed their diabetes entirely.

Just like migraine, diabetes was once thought to be a chronic and lifelong condition. The only real option was a drug to possibly lessen the symptoms and damage. Results like those above from the ketogenic diet weren't supposed to be possible. And yet....

Like I said earlier, we still have so much to learn.

Mental Health. Given the known neurophysiological similarities amongst seizures, migraines, and bipolar disorder, and given that ketones exert special effects on the brain, it's perhaps no surprise that it improves psychological well being. Research remains very early, but practitioners all over are employing a ketogenic diet. Just like with migraines and diabetes, the diet delivers results far better than anything else, allowing patients to come off of unpleasant drugs they'd been on for years or decades.

Areas where it is being investigated and used include anxiety disorders, major depression, bipolar, and autism spectrum disorders.

Alzheimer's, Parkinson's, and other neurodegenerative disorders. Virtually every chronic disease affecting the brain may benefit from a ketogenic diet - Alzheimer's and Parkinson's happen to be the most common and widely researched.

As I've mentioned, I already consider periodically adopting a ketogenic diet to be fundamental to preventing chronic disease of the brain. But there is now a growing body of evidence that nutritional ketosis can halt or even reverse the progression of neurodegenerative diseases like Alzheimer's and Parkinson's. For obvious reasons, this is an area of intense interest, one you're guaranteed to hear much more about in the coming years.

Autoimmune and Inflammatory Illnesses. The keto-genic diet reduces inflammation in multiple ways, both direct and indirect. Even viewed conservatively, this means it could be transformative for autoimmune conditions where the immune system attacks parts of the body.

But when we consider that inflammation is a signature of virtually every chronic disease of our time, then it becomes plausible to think that there's virtually no condition that it would not benefit.

Aging. Researchers in the field of aging have become increasingly excited about the possibility that ketosis can slow the aging process itself, irrespective of its impact on chronic disease. Recent studies in animals have shown that those who are fed a ketogenic diet at least part of the time live longer than those fed a standard diet.

Mental and Physical Performance. Those who push their brains and bodies to the height of performance are always looking for a competitive edge, which the ketogenic diet offers. In fact, its popularity has been accelerated by many high-profile athletes who are using a ketogenic diet to improve their athletic performance and their resilience, **so that they can perform better for longer.**

Even this cursory overview demonstrates that virtually every major category of illness appears to benefit from a ketogenic diet. And you can be sure that in the coming years, this list will continue to grow, as well our understanding of how to best use nutritional ketosis as a therapeutic weapon.

Perhaps this is a good time to point out that, while many people come to keto because of a specific problem they want to solve, they often stay keto because of the way they *feel* in ketosis. In addition to the many therapeutic benefits I've mentioned, for many ketosis just makes life....better. Better mood, more energy, clearer thinking, better sleep, and simply an increase in general well being.

So as exciting as its many potential therapeutic indications are, the significant impact of nutritional ketosis on quality of life may be equally transformative.

If you have someone in your life that you'd like to share this research with, you can find it (along with links to specific research studies) at ketoformigraine.com/research.

KEYS FROM CHAPTER 7:

1) There's reason to believe that the ketogenic diet could be used in the treatment of virtually every chronic disease of our time, from cancer to diabetes to autoimmune illness to dementia to mental illness.

2) As exciting as its potential as a therapeutic tool is, we should also not overlook the value of its impact on quality of life.

CHAPTER 8: 9 MYTHS ABOUT KETO

WHAT YOU'LL LEARN IN THIS CHAPTER: *In the wild west of the web, myths and misconceptions about keto abound, threatening all of your hard won progress. In this chapter, we'll cover some of the most common myths you're likely to encounter in the wild, wild west of the web.*

As bizarre as it seems, nutrition has become like politics and religion. Many have chosen sides and have closed their minds to other points of view.

Which is odd, not to mention unfortunate, for something that's at least supposedly based on science.

You don't see this happening in sciences like physics or chemistry. Friendships aren't ended by debates over the gravitational constant or the molecular weight of Boron.

But the health value of meat? Or the necessity of grains in a person's diet? Them's fightin' words!

What happened here?

Much of how we got here has to do with how nutritional research has been conducted over the last several decades.

In the sciences like chemistry and physics, we acquire knowledge through direct, controlled experimentation.

But the edifice of knowledge about nutrition, including the guidelines we were given about what we should and should not eat, was constructed out of much flimsier stuff. Because of that, many voices are now calling for a complete overhaul, arguing that what we really need is one big do-over. We are undoubtedly in the midst of a big correction phase in the field of nutrition.

In the meantime, you will encounter myths, many of which will be strongly held by those who espouse them.

You will encounter people who will try to persuade you to abandon your ways (usually they have no experience with the agony of migraines, and don't understand that you'd do just about anything to stop having them).

Some may be motivated out of legitimate concern — some out of a need to protect their interests or livelihood.

Others may envy your commitment and progress. It's human nature for others to feel as if the decisions you make in your own life are a judgment of theirs. Understand that their comments or criticisms have nothing to do with you.

You may even be met with concern from your doctors, many of whom are still way behind the curve when it comes to their knowledge and understanding of keto, and often decades behind when it comes to the science on cholesterol.

There are also keto rumors that spring up periodically and circulate the internet. Seldom is it clear where these come from. Russia, perhaps?

So, in order to fortify you against the most common keto myths and misconceptions, here's a round-up of the most common ones. Most of these are topics we've addressed in further depth elsewhere in the book, so I'm presenting them in short form so that you'll have the highlights here as an easy reference.

MYTH #1: ALL THAT FAT IS BAD FOR YOU.

Where this myth comes from: This of course comes from the belief that fat is bad for your cholesterol and will clog your arteries.

The details here make all the difference. Fat from vegetable and seed oils is bad for you.

But you won't be eating that.

As we discussed in Chapter 2, the hunch that saturated fat causes heart disease was never more than a hunch. A hunch that was never confirmed experimentally, and one that has now been roundly discredited.

The Reality: The ketogenic diet *will* change your blood cholesterol numbers - in ways that are linked to *lowering* your risk of clogged arteries, heart attacks, and strokes.

MYTH #2: KETOSIS IS DANGEROUS.

Where this myth comes from: The myth that ketosis was dangerous arose primarily because, when it was first rising in popularity, many health care providers would confuse it with a different condition known as "ketoacidosis." So, they'd hear mention that someone was voluntarily entering into ketosis, and they'd sound the alarm bells.

Most providers know better now, and no longer make this error of mistaken identity. Yet, the notion that ketosis can be dangerous lingers.

The Reality: Ketosis is a normal physiological state, like sleep.

For hundreds of thousands of years, humans have likely spent significant portions of their lives, if not the majority, in ketosis. In case you haven't noticed, we've done pretty okay as a species.

MYTH #3: YOU NEED CARBS IN YOUR DIET.

Where this myth comes from: This myth comes from the fact that there are cells of our body that require glucose (a carbohydrate) to stay alive. However, our bodies, being the wonders of nature that they are, can manufacture glucose just fine, through a process known as gluconeogenesis.

The Reality: There are essential amino acids we must get in our diet. There are essential fats we must get in our diet.

But there are no essential carbohydrates.

MYTH #4: YOU NEED CARBS TO KEEP YOUR BLOOD SUGAR UP.

Where this myth comes from: This one is a cousin of myth #3. And it comes from the combination of two misconceptions. One is that we must eat carbs to supply specific cells in our body with glucose. As just discussed, our body (specifically, our liver) is perfectly capable of manufacturing glucose to meet that need.

The second comes from a lack of awareness about how the brain uses ketones. There are still those who think that glucose is the only form of energy the brain can utilize, entirely unaware that ketones are an alternative energy source.

The Reality: The brain can make what glucose it needs, AND the brain can burn ketones for energy instead of glucose. Were that not true, this book wouldn't exist!

Furthermore, the longer you stay in ketosis, the more efficient your body becomes at producing ketones and the more efficient your brain becomes at using them. Those unfamiliar with the area of nutritional ketosis are usually mystified at how people in ketosis can have "dangerously low" blood sugars in the 40s or even 30s (in mg/dL) and still survive. How on earth is the brain able to remain conscious with so little fuel?

The answer, of course, is that the brain is using another fuel source - ketones. And feeling quite well doing so, thank you very much.

MYTH #5: YOU NEED GRAINS IN YOUR DIET.

Where this myth comes from: You can thank the food pyramid.

Actually, the set of guidelines under the "food pyramid" designation was first published in 1992. However, these were a visual recapitulation of the "Dietary Goals for the United States" document, which was drafted by a congressional committee on nutrition in 1977. Those recommendations were based almost entirely on the now-discredited Diet-Heart Disease hunch I've previously discussed.

Since fat was the bogeyman, and humans had to get their energy from somewhere, then carbs became the only place we were left to turn. So the guidelines advised us to obtain most of our calories from cereal grains (including wheat, barley, rye, and rice).

After those guidelines were established, grains suddenly found themselves vaulted to the top of the healthy food list. Why? Because they were the foundation of the pyramid. Chalk up another victory for circular reasoning!

So this entire idea that whole grains are the quintessential health food didn't come from any sort of rigorous scientific analysis, but rather from an accident of history.

The Reality: If we simply compare the nutritional content of grains with other nutritious foods like meat, organs, and non-starchy plants, we find there's no contest.

Consider one slice of (healthy!) whole wheat bread.

From a macronutrient standpoint, it contains a lot of carbohydrate, a little bit of protein, and hardly any fat. Yet, the protein is of low quality, as it is low in essential amino acids. Furthermore, some of the proteins that it does contain are ones known to damage the lining of our intestines.

Not looking good so far.

From a micronutrient standpoint, it contains hardly anything. Small amounts of iron, B-6, magnesium, and calcium. Yet, it also contains nutrient inhibitors and anti-nutrients that interfere with the absorption of those micronutrients. So it has few micronutrients to begin with, and even fewer that we can absorb.

Looking even worse.

On top of that, it comes with substances known to disrupt our guts, immune system, and blood-brain barrier.

Yikes!

So, nutritionally, the only thing it has going for it is that it is high in carbohydrates, and thus is a good source of energy. The problem is, to consume enough grains to meet your nutritional needs, you'd need to eat way more energy than you need. Doing that would lead to the accumulation of excess fat, aka obesity. And it would lead to intestinal and systemic inflammation.

In other words, relying on grains as your primary caloric source would lead to all the chronic health problems that have been ballooning out of control ever since we began making grains the foundation of the human diet.

RIP, grains.

So any time anyone tells you that your diet should include grains, or that you can't eliminate an entire food group from your diet, simply ask them this question: "what is there in grains that I can't get in greater amounts from other whole foods?"

Be prepared for an awkward silence.

MYTH #6: KETOSIS CAN INTERFERE WITH MEDICATIONS AND BE "DANGEROUS."

Where this myth comes from: Russia?

Seriously, this one popped out of nowhere one day and has been recurring periodically ever since. Nobody can cite a source for it other than the "internet" (aka the "myth-making machine").

The Reality: Dietary changes can indeed impact the metabolism of medications. So will exercise. Or sleeping in. Or waking up early. So will losing or gaining weight.

Yet, have you heard any warnings about the dangerous interaction of exercise, changing sleep habits, or weight loss with your medications?

Yes, any time you make significant changes to the way you live your life, it can impact how a given dose of medication affects you. It's always reasonable for anyone on chronic medications for chronic conditions to discuss major changes with their prescribing doctor (whether that doctor will be able to provide informed advice is a whole different ball of wax!).

These conversations are most important for those who are on specific medications where small changes in dosing can have an outsized effect on you (a "narrow therapeutic window," in technical terms). Often these are drugs where the level in your blood is being checked periodically.

As we've discussed, we already have evidence that a ketogenic diet can work wonders for diabetes. This means that, over time, a diabetic on a ketogenic diet will likely require less and less blood sugar lowering medication. Given that the ketogenic diet appears to have a favorable impact on a multitude of other conditions, this same medication-sparing effect will likely be seen in those as well. These, of course, are welcome changes, and certainly not something we'd wish to avoid!

MYTH #7: YOU'RE ONLY LOSING WATER WEIGHT ON KETO.

Where this myth comes from: The haters.

Seriously, though, it is true that carbohydrates cause us to retain water. Some refer to this as "bloating," or the "carb bloat." Apparently, models and actors have known about this phenomenon for decades.

This is why during the transition to keto you will urinate more. You are losing some of that excess water.

Those who are envious of your shrinking waistline may stretch this truth, claiming that all losses on keto are from water and that you'll gain all of it back as soon as you stop.

The Reality: The water losses are short term. Yes, some of the decline in those scale numbers in the first few days of keto is from water loss. But the body soon finds a new equilibrium, and those losses stop.

And, as we've discussed, other than complete fasting, keto is arguably the single best way to stimulate the loss of body fat. So you can rest assured that those losses are coming from where you want them to. Not that you were worried. Cause you know that haters gonna hate.

MYTH #8: A KETOGENIC DIET LEADS TO VITAMIN DEFICIENCIES

Where this comes myth from: I just saw this one today, as I was putting the final touches on this book! As if to prove my point, it comes from an article posted on a website for a to-remain-nameless movie that promotes a plant-based diet.

The Reality: While it's entirely possible to eat a version of a ketogenic diet that's nutrient-poor, virtually anyone who is moving from the standard Western to a ketogenic diet will be significantly improving the nutrient quality of their diet. This is especially true of a plan like *Keto for Migraine*, which sticks to eating human food.

The vast majority of our nutritional powerhouses have either zero or trivial amounts of carbohydrates and can be eaten liberally on a ketogenic plan, including our superstars of nutrient density: eggs, shellfish, organ meats, and greens.

MYTH #9: THERE IS ONE VERSION OF A KETOGENIC DIET

Where this myth comes from: If you view the ketogenic diet as nothing more than a way of eating that stimulates the production of ketones, then from that perspective, all ketogenic diets are the same.

The Reality: If there's one point I've hammered home more any other, it's that there is no such thing as a single ketogenic diet. And it makes no sense whatsoever to talk about the ketogenic diet as if it is one diet.

Yet, those who, for whatever reason, are threatened by the popularity of keto will *always* talk about the ketogenic diet as if it is one thing. Why? Because acknowledging that there are countless versions of it leaves nothing to attack. Nuance is the enemy of propaganda.

So if you come across anyone who talks as if the ketogenic diet is one single thing, walk briskly in the other direction.

KEYS FROM CHAPTER 8:

You will undoubtedly encounter efforts -fueled by less-than savory motivations - to besmirch the reputation of keto. While the myths covered in this chapter represent some of the most common mistruths spread in the keto-defamation project, I'm certain there will be many more. The knowledge you have acquired in this book should allow you to decipher fact from fiction.

CHAPTER 9: "FREQUENTLY ASKED QUESTIONS" ABOUT KETO FOR MIGRAINE

WHAT YOU'LL LEARN IN THIS CHAPTER: Here, I will address some commonly asked questions about the ketogenic diet and its use for migraines. Some of these topics are discussed elsewhere in the book but are important enough to warrant reiterating.

Also, if you're like me, it's highly improbable that you'll remember something after reading it once. Repetition is the friend of memory. So, I'd encourage you to read through this chapter even if you don't have any of these questions yet.

Q: What sweeteners do you recommend in place of sugar?

A: The short answer: I don't recommend using sweeteners for a multitude of reasons.

The long answer....so there was a time when I was young and naive and still relatively new to this keto thing, where I would recommend certain sweeteners to use in place of sugar.

Many migraineurs are rightly apprehensive about sugar substitutes. Some artificial sweeteners - Aspartame in particular - are known migraine triggers. Aspartame is an artificial sweetener, meaning it's a chemical made in a food lab. And chemicals made in food labs are best avoided by migraineurs (I'd argue they're best avoided by *everyone*).

In recent years, a host of other "natural" sweeteners have emerged as alternatives. I place natural in quotes here because these are really compounds isolated from plants. You certainly can't find them in isolated powder form in nature. That requires some extra bits of processing.

The most well known of the natural sweeteners (at this time) is probably Stevia, which is extracted from the Stevia Rebaudiana plant. Other "natural" sweeteners include erythritol and xylitol.

These have an advantage over sugar in that, while our brain perceives them to be as sweet as (or even sweeter) than sugar, they do not raise blood sugar levels. And they have fewer calories per gram than sugar (Stevia having zero calories), so are less likely to be fattening.

They also don't appear to pose any health risks.

So why do I not advise using them?

Because they actually make kicking the sugar habit harder.

For millennia now we humans have been monkeying with our food to make it ever tastier and tastier. We first did this when we began farming fruits and vegetables, selecting out the sweetest ones in each generation so that we continued to breed sweeter and sweeter plant foods. Many of our modern-day fruits and vegetables are orders of magnitude sweeter than the ones available to our hunting and gathering ancestors.

It's estimated that the sweetest fruits our wild ancestors had access to had the sweetness equivalent to a modern-day carrot. Think about that for a minute - for over 2 million years, the sweetest thing most humans would ever eat had the sweetness of a carrot.

Things got much worse in the industrial revolution with our ability to produce and refine sugar in mass quantities, and the emergence and widespread popularity of packaged convenience foods. Anyone who's read the labels of virtually every packaged food in the grocery store knows that the most common first ingredient is sugar.

So, for a few millennia, we've collectively been feeding an ever-growing addiction to sugar. That's been terrible for our collective health.

Not only has our excessive sugar consumption fed our growing epidemic of obesity and all its related diseases, but it has created an altogether unhealthy relationship with food.

Consider this: when you eat something that tastes really, really good, what are you liable to think about that food? Do you think that it's probably really good for you, or really bad for you?

Really bad, right?!

Pause for a moment to think how ridiculous that is.

What you're concluding here is that your brain, the most intelligent and sophisticated machine in the known universe, is screaming out for you to eat more of something that will hasten *its own death*.

To highlight the absurdity of this scenario, imagine you walk up to a campfire. As you approach, you begin feeling the heat of the flames. As you get closer, your skin gets hotter and hotter. At some point, it becomes unpleasant. Go far enough, and the pain will become unbearable. Virtually nobody would voluntarily walk into a burning flame, because the sensations their brain is generating will stop them from doing so.

And why does the brain generate those unpleasant sensations as we near the flames of a burning fire? Because catching fire is extraordinarily bad for your health!

Getting too close to fire feels bad. Moving away from it after getting too close feels good.

The sensations our brain generates exist for one reason - to ensure that we survive another day.

When our brain gives us pleasurable sensations, it's a signal that we're doing something good for us that we should keep doing. When it gives us unpleasant sensations, it's a signal that we're doing something harmful that we should stop doing.

Imagine if we extended our attitude about food to other sensations. In the case of the fire, we'd think, "I'm getting more and more uncomfortable the closer I get to this flame. I guess catching myself on fire must be good for me."

How in the world then did we reach this absurd situation with food where this got turned entirely upside down?

Because of sugar.

Our brain didn't evolve in the world of added sugar, and definitely not in the world of processed foods with tasty lab-made chemicals. Our brains' system for detecting whether something we eat is good for us - the system that registers that evaluation in the form of taste sensations - was not designed in a world full of refined sugar and Frankenfoods.

It's actually worse than that. Because in the wild, it was smart for us to eat something sweet. That would've primarily been ripened fruit that was only going to be edible for a day or so. Eating it right away before it went bad was a wise decision.

Those taste circuits serve us well in a world where sugar is scarce and only available in wild fruits and vegetables.

Problem is, over the last few millennia, we've been engineering our food to maximize sweetness, hijacking our brain's reward system that guides us on what to eat. This is how we find ourselves in the bizarre situation in which our brain tells us to eat more of a food that will hasten its own death!

The enormous upside of all this is that, once you stop hijacking your brain's reward system, you can restore a normal relationship with food. And all it takes is just to eat human food!

Only eating human food restores our brain's food feedback system to its rightful state, so that when it gives us a signal that something is super tasty, we can trust it to mean we're on the right track! **A juicy steak is delicious because a juicy steak is one of the most nutritious things we can put into our bodies.** That's because steaks have been part of the human diet for a very long time.

I've said many times that I enjoy eating so much more now than I ever did before. And I haven't had a doughnut, or bread, or a soft drink, or any of the foods that I used to consider "treats" in nearly a decade.

I eat what tastes great, secure in the knowledge that my brain is no longer being deceived.

Getting back to the original question, the reason I no longer advocate using sugar substitutes to sweeten foods is because doing so perpetuates the problem we're trying to escape. It obscures the natural flavors of the foods we're eating and is hijacking the taste centers of our brain, just like sugar does.

Furthermore, it makes us continue to crave things that taste sweet. It perpetuates the addiction to sweetness that was instigated by sugar, and so only prolongs suffering. Virtually everyone I've ever worked with who once thought themselves sugar addicts are surprised and amazed at how quickly the sugar cravings fade once it's eliminated from the diet.

So those are all the theoretical reasons why I no longer advise sweeteners.

Perhaps the most compelling reason is that I've seen what works and what doesn't. I and so many others have seen the same story play out more times than we can count - those who cut out sugar and ditch sweeteners altogether do great.

Ultimately, it's just about taking the surer route to success.

Q: It's been a couple of weeks, and I'm not showing ketones. Is there anything I can do?

A: While most people will begin to show ketones in their urine after a few days of eating this way, it's possible you may not. So first of all, don't worry.

Many different factors influence how fast the body begins producing ketones after adopting a ketogenic diet, which accounts for the variability in how long it takes to reach ketosis from one person to the next. And there are a few things you can do to accelerate the transition to ketosis.

1) Reduce daily carbohydrate intake, if possible. As discussed, most folks will produce ketones when carbs are restricted to between 20 and 50 grams per day. So, if you've been hovering closer to 50 grams, it's worth dropping down to 20 grams, or even under 20 grams.

Remember, while we humans must have protein and fat in our diet (to consume the essential amino acids and fats our bodies require), we do not need carbs.

2) Use Time Restricted Eating (TRE). "Time Restricted

Eating" is just a fancy term for only eating within a specific time during a 24 hour day. You do this by choosing an "eating window," which are the hours between which you will eat.

Whenever possible, it's also best to choose a time when your eating window opens. This will also determine the time your eating window closes. For example, if I choose a 10-hour eating window that starts at 8 am, then that means I will eat between the hours of 8 am and 6 pm. My fasting window, or the time within which I don't eat (drinking water is perfectly fine), will be 14 hours, between the hours of 6 pm and 8 am.

One of the cues our bodies use for deciding when to start ramping up its keto machinery is fasting. In fact, ketosis likely evolved as a strategy for us to continue to thrive during periods where we were without food for an extended time.

With the TRE strategy, you don't change anything about what you're eating, only when you're choosing to do so. A window of 10 to 12 hours is an excellent place to start. Give it a week. If you see ketones by then, great. If not, try shrinking the window a couple of hours for another week. And so on.

3) Get active. The more metabolically flexible you are, the faster you will transition into ketosis after restricting carbs to the ketogenic range. This is one reason why the first transition to ketosis takes the longest, because it's usually going to be the time when most people are the least metabolically flexible (because of eating the typical high-carb diet).

So, anything that improves metabolic flexibility will also accelerate the transition to keto. It turns out that physical activity is a great way to do just that. Exercise doesn't help people lose weight because it "burns calories," it helps because it improves metabolic flexibility.

The more you exercise, the better your cells become at burning stored fat when you need it, which means you're able to supply more of your energy through the burning of stored body fat than with food. And being better at burning stored body fat also means you'll hasten the transition to keto.

How much physical activity do we need to reap these benefits? Moderate aerobic activity for 30 minutes 3 times per week plus one session of resistance training has been shown to restore the cell's fat-burning abilities.

All that being said, if you're feeling good and making progress, even if you're not showing ketones, it's perfectly fine to keep doing what you're doing! As discussed, many of the benefits of eating this way are entirely unrelated to ketones themselves.

Q: Should I take "exogenous ketones" to increase the amount of ketones in my body and brain? Can I take them instead of eating a ketogenic diet?

A: This question is a perfect illustration of the difference between holistic and reductionist thinking, and how thinking holistically is so critical to making good health decisions.

Asking this question makes perfect sense if you have a reductionist approach to human health. Remember that in the reductionist approach, we're trying to break biology down to its finer constituents, in hopes of finding the *one pill* or supplement that we can take to fix what ails us. Searching for the silver bullet.

So, if the mission of a ketogenic diet is to produce ketones, then why not just bypass all the "hassle" of changing your diet and just pop some ketones in your mouth?!

First, for those who've never heard of an exogenous ketone, let me back up and explain what we're talking about here.

As discussed, *nutritional* ketosis occurs when the liver begins producing the ketone bodies acetoacetate and beta-hydroxy-butyrate and releasing them into the bloodstream. When our body is producing ketones, as they are here, they are known as "endogenous" ketones. In nutritional ketosis, we are making our own ketones.

In the past few years, as the ketogenic diet's popularity has surged, a new class of supplements has hit the market known as "exogenous" ketones. The difference here is that these are ketones that you ingest (typically in a powdered form that you mix into liquid), and are then absorbed into the bloodstream. Here, we're no longer making our own supply of ketones. We've outsourced the job to make life easier.

Sounds pretty good, eh?

First and foremost, this is *not* the same as nutritional ketosis. It is true that in both instances, ketones are floating around in the bloodstream, but the similarities end there. As we've discussed, many other changes are happening in the body when we adopt a ketogenic diet, many of which likely contribute to the benefits of the diet. **You get none of those benefits when you take exogenous ketones.**

Additionally, while nutritional ketosis is a natural physiologic state that humans have been in and out of for millions of years, exogenous ketones are entirely new. As a species, **we have no evolutionary experience with adding ketones to our body that we did not make,** which significantly increases the potential risks.

Some have also asked whether taking exogenous ketones during a migraine could be helpful as an abortive strategy. This is also something I would avoid and would predict to make migraines *worse*.

Why? Remember that migraines feed on an energy surplus. By ingesting ketones, we're essentially adding excess energy to the brain. While ketones are a cleaner form of energy than sugar, it is energy nonetheless, and in that regard, increases the likelihood of provoking The Beast.

The one scenario where these would be a reasonable option would be to reduce the transitional symptoms when first adopting a ketogenic diet (i.e., avoiding the "keto flu"). As discussed in chapter 4, one reason we experience those transitional symptoms is that the body is still gearing up what it needs to produce ketones and utilize them for energy. Exogenous ketones could help meet energy demands until that gearing up process is complete.

However, coconut and MCT oil can also provide an additional source of energy during that time. And they have the advantage of being time tested, less expensive, and better-tasting. So there's no real reason to choose exogenous ketones instead.

So is there any situation where taking exogenous ketones makes sense? The place where exogenous ketones may have a role is in athletic performance. Like the glucose gels that have long been a staple supplement in endurance sports, exogenous ketones can be taken before or during competitions to boost energy and improve stamina. And the research thus far has shown that they are helpful when used for that purpose.

Bottom line, given that we already have everything we need to reap incredible benefits from nutritional ketosis, **it's hard to justify adding in an unproven and potentially risky intervention to the mix.**

Q: Should I count the net or total grams of carbs?

A: If you do find yourself counting carbs at some point in this process, you will almost certainly wonder at some point whether to count *total* carbs or *net* carbs.

What am I talking about, you ask?

Carbohydrates refer to a class of macronutrients and can come in different forms.

The sugar in the sprinkles on top of a donut is a carbohydrate, as is the starch in the donut's batter.

What carbohydrate molecules have in common is that they are all compromised of carbon, oxygen, and hydrogen atoms combined in a specific ratio ("carbohydrate" is another way of saying "hydrated carbon."). But they come in many different shapes and sizes, and that shape and size significantly changes how they interact with our body.

Table sugar, which is part of the class of "simple sugars," is digested quickly. Starch, a complex carbohydrate found in many plants, takes a bit longer to digest.

And then there are other carbohydrates, like cellulose, that humans can't digest at all. When eaten, cellulose passes through the body undigested.

If you were to eat pure cellulose, it would have no impact on ketosis. Even though it's a carbohydrate, none of the sugar molecules can enter your bloodstream.

Many foods have a mix of different kinds of carbohydrates, including some that we can digest, and others we can't (usually a smaller proportion). These undigestable carbs are typically referred to as *fiber*.

So if you only wanted to track the carbs in food that will be absorbed into the body (assuming complete digestion), you'd subtract the amount of fiber from the total carbs in any food that you eat. You'll sometimes find this has already been done for you on food labels and provided under the term "net carbs."

Knowing this, your next question is whether or not to count

total or net carbs if you are counting carbs. My answer: it really doesn't matter. I and others have found that while this difference matters in theory, **in practice, it doesn't matter much.**

What's more important, in my opinion, is to choose one method and then be consistent. As mentioned, there's significant variability from one person to the next as to the degree of carbohydrate restriction needed to stimulate ketone production. So your primary objective when tracking carbs is to find your threshold, and you can do that effectively whether you're using total or net carbs.

When I track carbs, I track total carbs, mainly because I find it simpler.

Q: Is it ok to eat all my carbs in one meal or should I spread them out?

A: When it comes to the impact that carbs have on the body, it turns out that context matters quite a bit. In addition to the type of carbohydrate they are (simple or complex, fiber, etc.) when we eat them and what we eat them with makes a big difference in how they impact us. This is one of many reasons why different people have different carbohydrate thresholds for maintaining ketosis.

There are two main things to keep in mind here. The first is that it's best to avoid eating your carbs by themselves. For example, there are roughly 35 grams of carbs in a baked potato. If your carb target is 50 grams per day, then you could eat that potato and still be under your daily allotment.

However, eating that potato by itself would have a very different effect on your physiology than eating it as part of a more substantial mixed meal ("mixed" meaning it contains protein and fat). The former approach would lead to a much greater rise in blood sugar than the latter.

So the ideal strategy here is to first and foremost avoid eating your carbs all at once, by their lonesome, outside of the context of a mixed meal. And even better is to spread the carb allotment over the course of the day.

Q: What are good keto snacks?

A: I'll give you some snacking ideas along those lines in a sec, but I'd be remiss if I didn't take this opportunity to try to help re-frame your thoughts around snacking in general.

Snacks and snack foods are a modern invention, heavily pro-moted by the makers of packaged and processed convenience foods (and perhaps not coincidentally, it's these same foods that make us carbohydrate dependent and in need of those snacks in the first place!).

Snacking, and even our three-meals-a-day routine, were not a part of our ancestors' lifestyles. They are both artifacts of culture, and of the aforementioned carb dependency that the standard Western high-carb diet produces.

We humans do not require three meals a day, and certainly not three meals a day *plus* snacks! Remember, we are quite good at storing fat, precisely so that we can easily go extended times be-tween eating when the circumstances call for it - provided we're eating the foods we humans were meant to eat.

And remember that our goal isn't just to stimulate ketosis, but to also eat a diet *that's appropriate for a human*. Which also means returning to the eating patterns of our ancestors, who were not snackers.

That being said, as we've discussed, there is an adjustment phase between the time you embark on a ketogenic diet, and the time you've adapted to producing and burning ketones.

Once that adaptation kicks in, it typically leads to a surge in energy levels, thanks to the body's ability to mobilize and burn its stored body fat. This improvement in energy utilization results in the ability to go longer between meals, and often eliminates altogether the ravenous hunger so commonly experienced by those on a traditional high-carbohydrate diet. At that point, you will likely lose the desire to snack.

Before those adaptations have kicked in, however, there may be a short period where you do still get hungry between meals. What to do, then? Here are a few ideas:

Heat some leftovers. Leftovers are by far the best option (it just requires that you have leftovers). And here's where removing the concept of "snack foods" is helpful. Rather than thinking of a snack as its separate category, just think of it as a miniaturized version of your meals.

Super satisfying, nutrient-dense foods. Another way to handle this scenario is to use it as an opportunity to eat the most nutrient-dense foods around, ones loaded with healthy fats and proteins, along with a cornucopia of essential nutrients that many modern humans are lacking. Because of this, they also tend to be the most satisfying foods we can eat - so if you are going to "snack," let's make it count. The three superstars here are:

> **1) Hard-boiled (or deviled) eggs.** Not only are eggs nature's best snack, but they're also arguably the single best food a human can eat. High in healthy proteins and fats, and loaded with nutrients. This is also why they're so satiating (and feel free to prepare the eggs any way you like - hard-boiling transforms the egg into its most snack-able, grab-n-go form).

> **2) Sardines.** Also a contender for one of the most nutritious

foods a human can eat, and a source of nutrients that most modern humans don't get enough of. I prefer the ones from Wild Planet (link in the supplemental guide), and I like to dip them either in hot sauce or mustard.

3) Liverwurst. My favorite way to eat liver, along with other organ meats, is in the form of liverwurst (my favorite kind, which you can order online, is linked in the supplemental guide).

Eat more food at mealtimes. We only get energy from two sources - the energy we eat and the energy we store. And until your fat and ketone burning machinery has fully kicked in, you'll likely just need to increase the amount of energy you eat.

Add more fat to your meals. Liberal use of healthy fats like olive oil and butter, besides being delicious, will also add energy to your meals, provide more substrates for ketosis, and stimulate that fat burning machinery (you'll find our favorite olive oil for everyday use in the supplemental guide).

Sparkling mineral water. Unless I'm super hungry, a glass of sparkling mineral water is often enough to curb my hunger for another hour or two.

Unfortunately, the internet is full of all manner of keto snack foods that aren't part of the *Keto for Migraine* plan, and that can inadvertently end up reinforcing the very habits we're trying to break. Stick to the guidelines presented here, and avoid unwittingly sabotaging all your hard work!

Q: If I cheat and knock myself out of ketosis, will that unravel all my hard work?

A: Short answer: not at all.

Long answer: Imagine that zippers have become the latest craze, so you decide to start a zipper company.

You build a zipper factory. You buy all of your equipment, assemble it, hire workers, train them on how to use it, and so on.

In those early phases, a lot is happening to get you ready to make zippers. You've spent a lot of money and done a lot of work, but you haven't made a single zipper yet.

This is you when you're first starting a ketogenic diet.

Eventually, you're making zippers. Things are a little slow at first as people learn what they're doing, and you figure out the kinks in the system. Over the first few weeks, your production of zippers steadily increases.

At some point, your zipper production stabilizes. Over time, you continue to refine your processes and become even more efficient at making zippers.

This is you once you've become "keto-adapted."

Then, the button craze hits, and the demand for zippers plummets. To save money, you stop zipper production for a while.

This is you when you're knocked out of ketosis.

Now, are you in the same situation you were in before you ever built your zipper factory? Of course not, you still have all of your equipment and know-how ready to go.

If the demand for zippers goes up again, you can meet it.

Whether it's zipper business building or keto-adaptation, all that hard work doesn't disappear overnight.

WHERE TO GO NEXT

First of all, let me say thank you.

No, not for buying this book, though I do greatly appreciate it.

Thank you for giving me something far more valuable than money: your time. Time is, without a doubt, our most precious resource.

Thank you for the time you've taken to read this book.

As I said when we began this journey together, I wrote this book because this information is too important to keep to myself. Years ago, while suffering from an unrelenting week-long migraine, I said to myself that nobody should ever suffer like this. And I made a promise to myself to do everything in my power to create a future where that was true.

So thank you for the time you've taken to read. And even more, thank you for putting this into action. Over the past few years of building our Migraine Miracle community, I've been astounded at how words can change lives.

When I wrote *The Migraine Miracle* in 2013, I said it'd all be worth it if it changed just one person's life.

What ended up happening has exceeded my wildest dreams. More lives have been impacted than I could've possibly imagined.

And most of that hasn't been because of me, but because of people like you. People sharing this message. People experiencing results they never thought possible, and then feeling compelled as I did to get the word out.

But there is much more work to be done. There are still far more people who need to hear this message than have heard it.

So what next? Here are some ideas:

1) Keep it going!

You've made a commitment to your health by reading this book and putting it into action, and experienced what a holistic approach to health can do. Keep the momentum going.

This series will contain more about how to implement a holistic practice to slay The Beast, as well as to afford yourself the best possibility of living a long life well-lived.

2) Join our community.

First, be sure that you're part of our growing community. If you downloaded the Supplemental Guide to this book (ketoformigraine.com/guide), then you'll receive my email newsletter. If you're on Facebook, please join our group ("Dr. T's Migraine Miracle group").

If you haven't already, be sure to subscribe to the "Migraine Miracle Moment" podcast.

3) Join a Keto Blast challenge.

For the past several years, we've regularly held our 30-day Keto Challenges for our members of Migrai-Neverland (one of several regular challenges we do with members). Many have found the support and accountability of the group challenge, as well as the ability to ask me questions along the way, to be a vital component in their long-term success with keto.

To learn more about Migrai-Neverland along with all of our other resources for migraineurs, go to mymigrainemiracle.com/how-we-can-help.

4) Share with others.

If you want to help spread the word so that other migraine sufferers can find the relief they desperately need, the **best place to start is to leave a review of this book on Amazon.**

Beyond that, consider sharing your experiences with interested friends, coworkers, and family.

I am so profoundly grateful to all those in our community who've shared their incredible transformations with their doctors, in our Facebook group, and on the Migraine Miracle Moment podcast. There is nothing more powerful than hearing the story of someone who was once in your shoes.

You have made more of a difference than you will probably ever know, and you are all my heroes.

Made in the USA
San Bernardino, CA
24 February 2020